T0133443

The Obscure Sacroiliac Joint

This book summarizes contemporary basic science understanding of sacro-iliac joint anatomy, biomechanics, and disease with related changes in the joint. It provides insight into emerging and promising therapeutic options. Combining established concepts and recent findings on the sacroiliac joint, together with research advances made over the last 25 years, this illustrated text will appeal to pain therapists, orthopedic practitioners, spine surgeons, sacroiliac joint surgeons, physiotherapists, and general practitioners.

The Obscure Sacroiliac Joint

Insights into joint anatomy, biomechanics, etiology and the treatment of mechanical dysfunction

Edited by
Niels Hammer, MD, Dr. habil.

Authors
Julius Dengler, MD, Dr. habil.
Daisuke Kurosawa, MD
Amélie Poilliot, PhD
Jennifer Saunders, MBBS, PhD, FACSEP
Britt Stuge, PT, PhD

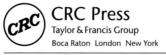

CRC Press
Taylor & Francis Group
Boca Raton London New York

CRC Press is an imprint of the
Taylor & Francis Group, an **informa** business

First edition published 2023
by CRC Press
6000 Broken Sound Parkway NW, Suite 300, Boca Raton, FL 33487–2742

and by CRC Press
4 Park Square, Milton Park, Abingdon, Oxon, OX14 4RN

CRC Press is an imprint of Taylor & Francis Group, LLC

© 2023 Taylor & Francis Group, LLC

ISBN: 978-1-032-39044-4 (hbk)
ISBN: 978-1-032-38706-2 (pbk)
ISBN: 978-1-003-34816-0 (ebk)

DOI: 10.1201/9781003348160

Typeset in Palatino
by Apex CoVantage, LLC

*Dedicated to patients and doctors who will
benefit from this book.*

Contents

Preface

Joints are designed for motion. This principle applies in particular to the musculoskeletal system. The technical concepts we use in engineering sciences are informed by the principles found in nature, especially within our own body. Our musculoskeletal system is designed for movement under a variety of static and dynamic scenarios, and the sacroiliac joint plays an important yet underestimated role in our daily activities. It has gained increasing interest as a source of pain over the last few years, owing to its common involvement in low back pain.

The sacroiliac joint functionally connects the spine and the pelvis. Despite the versatile function this joint must fulfill, it remains obscure to most of us for a lifetime. However, for those affected by its dysfunction, daily life is impaired to a significant extent. Contemporary research on sacroiliac joint anatomy, pathology, and treatment has so far been carried out by a small community of specialists, facing a growing body of widespread basic science and clinical data. A variety of new treatment strategies have evolved over the last decades, both non-surgical and surgical. Consequently, the reciprocal integration of basic science concepts on sacroiliac joint morphology, kinematics, and therapeutic advancements is challenged.

Our book aims to summarize contemporary basic science knowledge on sacroiliac joint anatomy, biomechanics, and disease with related changes in the joint, and to give insight into emerging and promising therapeutic options. It combines established concepts and recent findings on the sacroiliac joint, and research advances made over the last 25 years. The idea for this book was inspired by the work of Professor Rudolf Kissling. It is meant to complement the growing body of literature on surgical interventions to the joint provided by our research colleagues, partners, and friends in various parts of the world.

This book is equally addressed to our clinical colleagues, anatomists, and biomechanicists with interest on the topic. We have been able to attract several renowned experts in the field, including Dr. Amélie Poilliot (Switzerland), Associate Professor Jennifer Saunders (Australia), Dr. Britt

Stuge (Norway), Professor Julius Dengler (Germany), and Dr. Daisuke Kurosawa (Japan).

Andreas Bauer (Austria) illustrated most of the images in the book, and PD Dr. Hanno Steinke (Germany) has generously helped provide the plastinates showing the fine anatomy of the joint.

On behalf of all the authors,

Niels Hammer

Graz, Austria

Editor

Niels Hammer, MD, Dr. habil.
Gottfried Schatz Research Center
Division of Macroscopic and
    Clinical Anatomy
Medical University of Graz
Graz, Austria

Department of Orthopedic,
    Trauma, and Plastic Surgery
University of Leipzig
Leipzig, Germany

Division of Biomechatronics
Fraunhofer Institute for Machine
    Tools and Forming Technology
Dresden, Germany

Authors

Julius Dengler, MD, Dr. habil.
Department of Neurosurgery
Helios Clinic
and
Brandenburg Medical School
    Theodor Fontane
Campus Bad Saarow
Bad Saarow, Germany

Daisuke Kurosawa, MD
Department of Orthopedic Surgery
Japan Sacroiliac Joint and Low
    Back Pain Center
JCHO Sendai Hospital
Sendai, Japan

Amélie Poilliot, PhD
Anatomical Institute
University of Basel
Basel, Switzerland

**Jennifer Saunders, MBBS, PhD,
    FACSEP**
Sydney School of Medicine
University of Notre Dame
Sydney, Australia

Britt Stuge, PT, PhD
Division of Orthopaedic Surgery
Oslo University Hospital
Oslo, Norway

chapter one

Morphology of the Sacroiliac Joint

Amélie Poilliot and Niels Hammer

Contents

The sacroiliac joints form parts of two of three joints of the pelvic girdle. Located posteriorly, the joints are formed by the articulation of the iliac part of the innominate (coxal) bone with the corresponding side of the sacrum (Figure 1.1). The sacroiliac joint is composed of two distinct parts: an anterior diarthrotic and a posterior syndesmotic 'ligamentous' part (Figure 1.2). The anterior diarthrotic compartment is considered a 'true' articulation, where the complementary auricular surfaces of the ilium and sacrum unite. This region presents most of the classic features of a synovial joint (von Luschka, 1854; Albee, 1909; Brooke, 1923; Macdonald and Hunt, 1952; Bowen and Cassidy, 1981), thus forming the diarthrodial part of the joint. The posterior syndesmotic region is where the interosseous ligaments tether the sacropelvic surface of the ilium and with the sacral fossae and lateral sacral crest. Fatty tissue and small vessels are also present in this region, between the dense meshes of interosseous ligament (Sashin, 1930; Weisl, 1954; Puhakka et al., 2004; Poilliot et al., 2019a; Poilliot et al., 2020b).

DOI: 10.1201/9781003348160-1

1

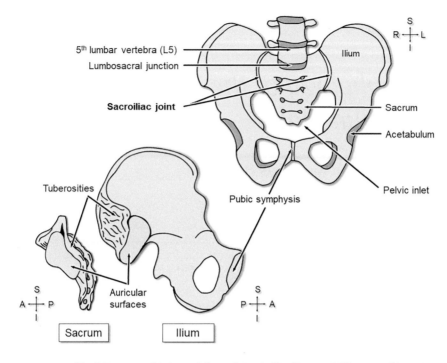

Figure 1.1 (Top) Bones and joints of the pelvic girdle. (Bottom) The sacroiliac joint articular surfaces on the ilium (right) and the sacrum (left). A: anterior, I: inferior, L: left, P: posterior, R: right, S: superior.

1.1   Embryology

Often classified as a diarthrosis with an amphiarthrodial function (Robert et al., 2009), the sacroiliac joint is arguably more complex in its classification. Embryologically, the anterior sacroiliac joint portion develops in the same way as other diarthrodial joints starting around the eighth week of gestation (Figure 1.3). Cavitation occurs later (tenth week in utero) and progresses less rapidly until the seventh month of gestation (Bellamy et al., 1983). Also, the joint does not cavitate uniformly as seen in other joints (Schunke and Bernard, 1938; Okumura et al., 2017). The posterior sacroiliac joint develops as a singular large collagenous ligament which will eventually develop into the interosseous ligament (Bowen and Cassidy, 1981).

1.2   Classification of the Sacroiliac Joint

With older age comes anticipated degenerative changes and a decrease in mobility reflecting features of an amphiarthrosis (Sashin, 1930; Bowen

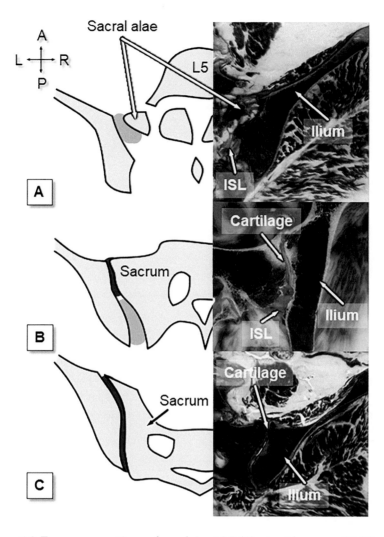

Figure 1.2 Transverse sections of a pelvis at L5 (A), at mid-sacrum S2 (B), and at S3/S4 (C) with the corresponding E12 plastinate on the right. On the left side, darker gray regions highlight the cartilaginous (synovial) portion, and the lighter gray regions show the ligamentous (syndesmotic) portion with the interosseous sacroiliac ligament (ISL). A: anterior, L: left, P: posterior, R: right.

and Cassidy, 1981). Therefore, it is difficult to accurately classify the sacroiliac joint. It presents diarthro-amphiarthrodial characteristics and its classification depends on the features used for the assessment (Walker, 1992; Poilliot et al., 2019b).

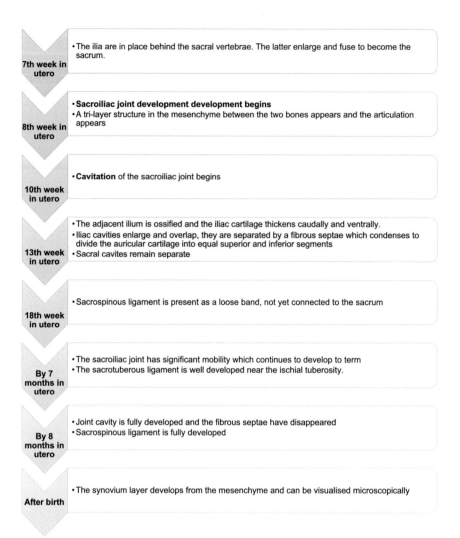

Figure 1.3 Embryological development of the sacroiliac joint and surrounding structures.

Source: Bellamy et al. (1983); Hayashi et al. (2013); Okumura et al. (2017).

The sacroiliac joint is uniquely different from other classic synovial joints. Its primary function is to provide stability to the pelvic girdle to allow the adequate transmission of the body weight to the hip bones (Fortin et al., 1999; Forst et al., 2006; Szadek et al., 2009; Hammer et al., 2019c; Kiapour et al., 2020), while at the same time providing enough movement to dissipate load peaks at the spinopelvic transition. This stability is achieved via a combination of morphological features, namely:

(1) The auricular surfaces which are covered with ridges and depressions providing a strong interlocking system between the ilia and the sacrum (Snijders et al., 1993; Puhakka et al., 2004; Forst et al., 2006),
(2) the dense ligamentous network surrounding the joint (Vleeming et al., 1997), and
(3) the muscles spanning from the sacroiliac joint (Vleeming et al., 1995a; Vleeming and Schuenke, 2019).

The combination of these features together is termed 'form and force closure', and allows the posterior pelvis to have the unique role of providing overall stability with some degree of movement. Naturally, the juxtaposition of seemingly opposite functions is the foundation of potential complications within the sacroiliac joint complex. The addition of other variables, including age, sex, and anatomical variation, complicates the joint's classification and its evolution during life as these features can affect the delicate equilibrium between stability and movement.

1.3 *Anthropological Aspects and Sexual Dimorphism of the Human Pelvis*

The human pelvis has evolved from quadrupedalism to bipedalism, requiring the pelvis to support a significant portion of the body weight under both static and dynamic situations. In conjunction to this, the female pelvis serves another fundamental purpose in parturition: it must be deformable enough to allow for the passage of the fetus. These two functions of the pelvis require conflicting anatomical needs and therefore lead to complications during childbirth (Trevathan, 1987). The female pelvis must retain an expanded birth canal (Figure 1.4), yet also remain narrow enough to allow efficient bipedalism (Tague and Lovejoy, 1986; Aulds, 2019). This has evolved into larger sacroiliac joint regions in bipedal mammals to provide more stability and support. Sexual dimorphism is well recognized, as appearing in both the anterior articular and posterior interosseous parts of the sacroiliac joint (İşcan and Derrick, 1984; Anastasiou and Chamberlain, 2013) having been shown that females have a larger joint than males (Poilliot et al., 2019a). Furthermore, there is a considerable difference in the ligaments between both sexes. No sex differences are evident until puberty, but thereafter the strength of the ligaments is sacrificed in females for increased mobility in preparation for pregnancy and labor (Bellamy et al., 1983; Hammer et al., 2009; Hammer et al., 2010; Steinke et al., 2010).

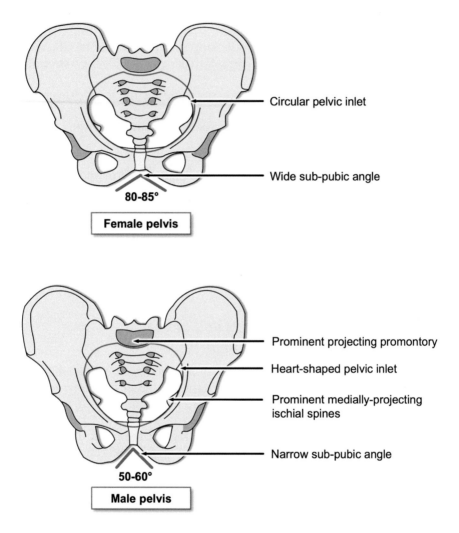

Figure 1.4 Sexual dimorphism of the human pelvis between biological males and females.

1.4   *Cartilage Anatomy*

The articular surface is covered with fibrocartilage on the ilium and hyaline cartilage on the sacral side (Schunke and Bernard, 1938; Resnick et al., 1975; Benneman, 1979; Paquin et al., 1983; Christ et al., 2001). The cartilage on the sacral side averages one to four millimeters in width and extends as a continuous layer attached within the joint cavity to the borders of the auricular surfaces (von Luschka, 1854; Albee, 1909; Brooke, 1923; Schunke and Bernard, 1938; Macdonald and Hunt, 1952; Puhakka et al., 2004). The iliac cartilage measures only a fraction of the thickness of the cartilage on the sacral side and does not fluctuate with age (von Luschka, 1854; Macdonald and Hunt, 1952; Bowen and Cassidy, 1981). In younger individuals, the sacral cartilage appears as smooth, light-gray or 'glistening' and the iliac side has a blueish tint with a striated or striped appearance. With age, both cartilages roughen and tarnish to a more yellow appearance (Luschka, 1854; Sashin, 1930; Macdonald and Hunt, 1952; Bowen and Cassidy, 1981; Dijkstra et al., 1989). These changes in cartilage surface seem to be related to an enhanced coefficient of friction, allowing for more effective load transfer in the upright stance. Although the features the cartilage surface presents would be considered osteoarthritic in other regions of the body, there is evidence that this change is unrelated to pathology but rather to functional adaptation.

1.5   Osseous Anatomy

At birth the sacroiliac joint is straight and parallel to the spinal column and gradually curves in a posterior direction and increases in width during childhood development. These changes are induced by mechanical forces related to bipedal gait (Bellamy et al., 1983). The osteology of the adult sacroiliac joint is variable. The second sacral vertebra is always involved in the articulation and the segments S1, S2, and S3 form the most common combination involved in the joint, while L4, L5, and S4 are occasionally involved. Some of this variation can be related to sexual dimorphism: that is, female pelves usually have fewer sacral segments than male pelves (Bellamy et al., 1983).

The auricular surfaces are pitted and ridged and interlock solidly to enhance stability and inhibit movement between the innominate and the sacrum (Snijders et al., 1993; Forst et al., 2006). The articular surface of the sacrum is more concave and larger in area than the convex iliac surface (Brooke, 1923; Sashin, 1930; Simkin et al., 1980). There is variation in the shape of the articulating surfaces of both the ilium and sacrum. The most common variant in shape is an accessory dorsal projection of the joint at the caudal end (Bellamy et al., 1983). The articular surface is formed of two 'limbs' assembled in variable crescent shapes, described as 'L', 'C', or sometimes 'V' shaped with a mean angle averaging between 93° and 100° (Brooke, 1923; Schunke and Bernard, 1938; Macdonald and Hunt, 1952; Waldrop et al., 1993; Rana et al., 2015; Postacchini et al., 2017; Casaroli et al., 2020). The shape of the auricular surfaces can be characterized into three morphology types (Jesse et al., 2017; Ou-Yang et al., 2017) (Figure 1.5):

- Type 1 is scone-shaped with a posterior border angle of > 160°
- Type 2 is auricle-shaped with a posterior border angle of 130–160°
- Type 3 is crescent-shaped with a posterior border angle of < 130°

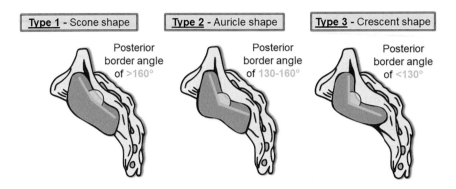

Figure 1.5 Classification of auricular surface shapes.

The angle is also reflective of the shape and volume of the interosseous ligaments, which are situated posterior to the auricular cartilage areas on both sides.

The variations observed frequently at the sacroiliac joint are likely to have an impact on function. Morphological differences of the sacroiliac joint from the 'typical healthy joint', which refers to the most frequent joint morphology, is depicted in Figure 1.6. The following morphological variations were reported in patients with no sacroiliac joint-related problems (Prassopoulos et al., 1999; Demir et al., 2007; El Rafei et al., 2018; Tok Umay and Korkmaz, 2020):

- accessory sacroiliac joints
- the iliosacral complex
- bipartite appearance/dysmorphic changes
- single semi-circular defects
- crescent-like iliac articular surface
- isolated synostosis
- small ossification centers of sacral wings

The most common anatomical variant of the sacroiliac joint are *accessory sacroiliac joints*. These are 'additional articular facets' within the syndesmotic region of the joint (Petersen, 1905; Seligman, 1935; Schunke and

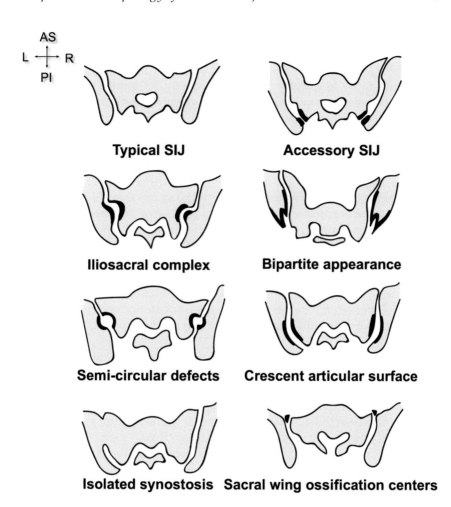

Figure 1.6 Examples of transverse sections of ilium and sacrum as can be found between S1 and S4 showing variation in joint morphology; these may occur in conjunction with one another. AS: anterosuperior, L: left, PI: posteroinferior, R: right, SIJ: sacroiliac joint.

Bernard, 1938; Trotter, 1940; Bakland and Hansen, 1984; Ehara et al., 1988; Valojerdy and Hogg, 1990; Walker, 1992; Prassopoulos et al., 1999; El Rafei et al., 2018; Cihan et al., 2020). Accessory joints are a result of the sinking and further rotation of the sacrum, which induces the development of accessory sacroiliac joints at places where the ligaments are attached and where the posterior superior iliac spine joins the sacrum (Seligman, 1935). The *iliosacral complex* morphology is an iliac projection inserting into a

sacral recess at the level of S1–S2 at the cranial posterior part of the posterior syndesmotic region or the inferior articular portion (Prassopoulos
et al., 1999; El Rafei et al., 2018; Tok Umay and Korkmaz, 2020). This variation occurs more frequently in females, mostly bilaterally between the
first and second sacral foramina. A *bipartite appearance* reflects dysmorphic
posterior iliac changes, more frequently reported in females, occurring in
approximately 30% of cases unilaterally and 70% bilaterally (El Rafei et al.,
2018). *Single semi-circular defects* in the articular surface occur in approximately 4% of people, mostly bilaterally (Prassopoulos et al., 1999). These
are more common in females at the posterior superior aspect of interosseous region with all cases found only on the sacral side (El Rafei et al.,
2018). *Crescent-like articular surfaces* are a bulged sacral surface appearance
which occurs in approximately 4% of patients, bilaterally and unilaterally.
It is more common in women than men with no relation to age. *Isolated
synostosis* was noted as unilateral involving the middle third of the right
sacroiliac joint at the level of the first sacral foramen occurring in less than
1% of cases. Finally, *small ossification centers* of the sacral wings appearing
as triangular osseous structures in the superior anterior region of the sacroiliac joint were found to occur in 0.6% of patients (Prassopoulos et al.,
1999).

The pelvic bone is an efficient structure, consisting of low-density trabecular bone covered in a layer of high-density cortical bone enabling it
to be a low-weight structure capable of withstanding high loads (Dalstra
and Huiskes, 1995). In healthy adults, the subchondral bone density distribution of the sacroiliac articular surfaces is highest in the superior and
anterior regions on the iliac side and in the anterior region on the sacral
side (Poilliot et al., 2020a, 2021), specifically around the S1–S2 anterior portion of the sacrum (Figure 1.7) (Ebraheim et al., 2000; Hoel et al., 2017).
Furthermore, the sacral side appears approximately half as dense than
its iliac counterpart at the anterior, central, and posterior portions of the
joint (McLauchlan and Gardner, 2002). Cortical thickness does not vary
between sexes nor with age, ranging from 0.5 to 2.3 millimeters thickness (Peretz et al., 1998). Regarding the subchondral bone architecture of
the sacroiliac counterparts, the sacral subchondral bone plate is thin with
trabecular spongiosa inserting into it at a right angle. The iliac bone, however, is thicker, with the trabecular spongiosa inserting into the bone plate
obliquely (Kampen and Tillmann, 1998).

1.6   Ligamentous Anatomy

The main stabilizers of the sacroiliac joint are presented by a dense
network of intrinsic and extrinsic ligaments, sometimes referred
to as 'capsular' and 'accessory ligaments' (Weisl, 1954; Cuppett and
Paladino, 2001).

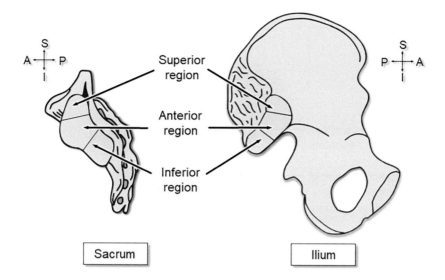

Figure 1.7 Regions of the sacral and iliac auricular surfaces. A: anterior, I: inferior, P: posterior, S: superior.

The group of intrinsic ligaments directly connects the sacrum with the ilium, surrounding the joint:

- anterior sacroiliac ligament
- interosseous ligament
- posterior sacroiliac ligament
- long posterior sacroiliac ligament (often referred to as part of the posterior sacroiliac joint ligament)

The group of extrinsic ligaments has no direct or incomplete contact with the joint:

- iliolumbar ligament
- sacrospinous ligament
- sacrotuberous ligament

Because the synovial anterior part of the joint is relatively flat, loaded stability cannot be achieved on the basis of bony interlocking alone, therefore, the extra-capsular ligaments must offer enough resistance to compensate the shear forces used in force closure (Vleeming et al., 1997).

The *anterior sacroiliac ligaments* stabilize the joint anteriorly as a thickening of the anterior and inferior parts of the fibrous joint capsule passing from the sacrum to the antero-medial border of the ilium (Figure 1.8)

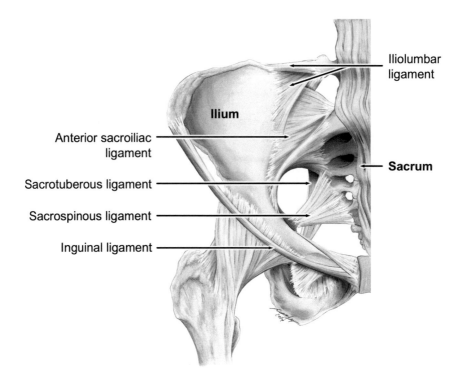

Figure 1.8 Ligaments of the sacroiliac joint (anterior view).

(Sashin, 1930; Weisl, 1954; Gerlach and Lierse, 1992; Puhakka et al., 2004; Steinke et al., 2010; Poilliot et al., 2019b). They consist of two to three sub-structures: the superior, middle, and inferior parts that spread in a fan-like shape from the anterior sacrum to the wing of the ilium (Hakim, 1937; Weisl, 1954; Gerlach and Lierse, 1992; Steinke et al., 2010; Poilliot et al., 2019b). The superior part arises from the ventral half of the lateral border of the sacral ala and continues to the adjacent medial border of the iliac fossa (Weisl, 1954). The thickness and width of the ligament increases at the pelvic brim while spreading along the ilium for 20 millimeters mingling with fibers from the iliolumbar ligament superiorly. On the anterior pelvic aspect, the inferior fibers attach laterally in a line at the first three sacral foramina converging together dorso-laterally forming the narrowest part of the greater sciatic notch (Weisl, 1954). The inferior part of the anterior sacroiliac ligament is continuous with the posterior, sacrospinous, and sacrotuberous liga-ments (Steinke et al., 2014). The inferior aspect of the sacral ala is entrapped between the ligaments, which may predispose the area to avulsion frac-tures in cases of pelvic injury (Steinke et al., 2014). The anterior sacroiliac ligaments are fenestrated and often very thin. Owing to these features, their load bearing functions is often challenged.

Posterior to the synovial part of the sacroiliac joint with its auricular surface, stability is enhanced via a thick network of ligament running through the posterior joint recess in various layers and directions. The deepest and most central layer is the large *interosseous* ligament which fills the syndesmotic joint space between the iliac and sacral tuberosities (Figure 1.9) (Rosatelli et al., 2006). Fibers have a dorso-lateral (cranial group) and cranial (caudal group) directionality from their sacral attachments. Each group has approximately 13 bundles of parallel fibers with the caudal group having longer and flatter fibers than the cranial group. Bundles insert into the retro-auricular regions of the sacrum and ilium in the cranial part of the joint (Steinke et al., 2010). Ventrally, the attachments are separated from the articular surface by a narrow strip of intra-capsular bone. Dorsally and cranially, they reach the lateral crest border of the sacral ala and run up to the crest and medial border of the iliac fossa (Weisl, 1954).

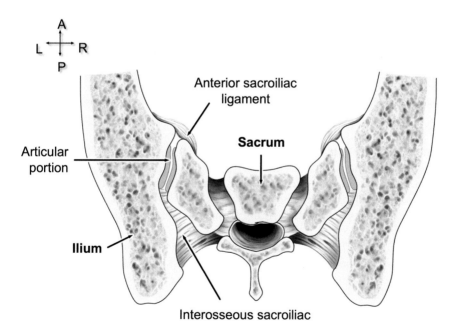

Figure 1.9 Transverse section of the sacroiliac joint. The posterior syndesmotic portion is filled with the interosseous sacroiliac ligament. In green is the cartilage of the anterior synovial portion of the joint. A: anterior, L: left, P: posterior, R: right.

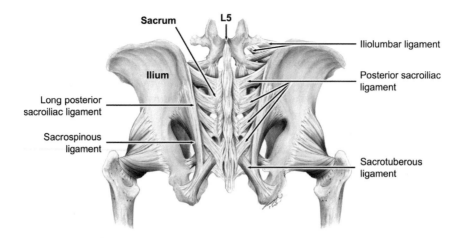

Figure 1.10 Posterior view at the posterior ligamentous complex of the sacroiliac joint.

The second layer includes the *posterior sacroiliac ligaments* which act as a posterior reinforcement of this same mass of ligamentous tissue and aid in counterbalancing counternutation (Figure 1.10) (Eichenseer et al., 2011; Kiapour et al., 2020). These ligaments run from the lateral sacral crest to the ilium, that is, posterior superior iliac spine (PSIS) and iliac tuberosity. Similar to the other intrinsic ligaments, the posterior sacroiliac ligaments also fan out dorso-laterally in various patterns to the adjacent bony structures in between these sites (Hakim, 1937; Weisl, 1954; Gerlach and Lierse, 1992; Poilliot et al., 2019b). It is located cranially and caudally to the articular space (Steinke et al., 2010) and its fibers merge with the anterior sacroiliac ligament superiorly (Poilliot et al., 2019b).

Lastly, the final layer of posterior ligaments situated most posteriorly and superficially is the *long posterior sacroiliac ligament* complex, which presents as a fibrous sheet running from the posterior superior iliac spine to the third or fourth lateral sacral tubercles (Figure 1.10) (Weisl, 1954; Vleeming et al., 1996; McGrath et al., 2009). The long posterior sacroiliac ligaments have been described as being formed of weak fascicles passing dorso-laterally from the superior articular process and from each of the posterior sacral tubercles to the inner lip of the iliac crest. Moreover, parallel fibers flattened dorso-ventrally running from the posterior border of the iliac bone (posterior superior iliac spine) to the inferior border of the lateral sacral crest and sacrotuberous ligament (Weisl, 1954; McGrath et al., 2009).

The most cranially situated of the extrinsic ligaments is the *iliolumbar ligament*. It is formed of one to four distinct ligament bands, but is most often described to be composed of bands (Figure 1.10) (Luk et al., 1986;

Uhthoff, 1993; Hanson and Sonesson, 1994; Basadonna et al., 1996; Rucco et al., 1996; Hartford et al., 2000; Hammer et al., 2010; Zoccali et al., 2016). An anterior band arises from the tip of the transverse process of L5 running dorso-laterally to the periosteum on the anterior margin of the iliac crest (Luk et al., 1986) in an infero-lateral direction indicating a torsion in its course (Hammer et al., 2010). The posterior band runs dorsally from L5 to the posterior margin of the iliac crest in a 'torsion manner' or a 'small cone' (Luk et al., 1986; Rucco et al., 1996; Hammer et al., 2010). It has been found to also arise from the lateral part of the dorso-inferior part of the L5 transverse process and inserts below the medial part of iliac crest on the anterior part of the iliac tuberosity. It is said to attach superiorly to its anterior counterpart or to the anterior margin of iliac crest (Hanson and Sonesson, 1994; Basadonna et al., 1996). Ligament attachments from L4 seem not to exist. They are often confused as being the epimysium of quadratus lumborum, which is situated in close proximity to the ligament and notably at L4 (Hammer et al., 2010).

Running between the sacrum, ischial spine, and ischial tuberosity there are the other two significant extrinsic ligaments: the sacrospinous and sacrotuberous ligament (Figure 1.11) (Hammer et al., 2009; Hammer

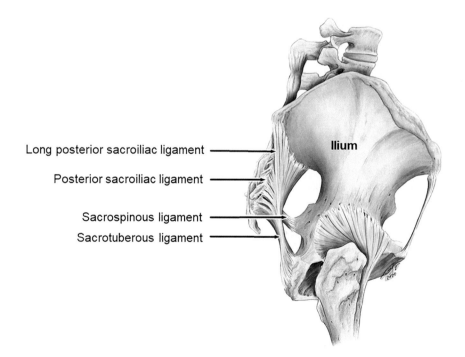

Figure 1.11 Lateromedial view of the pelvis and sacroiliac joint ligaments.

et al., 2013). The *sacrospinous ligament* arises from the antero-lateral surface of the last two sacral segments and the first coccygeal segment to the ischial spine (Sashin, 1930; Gerlach and Lierse, 1992) and the *sacrotuberous ligament* arises along a line running from the posterior inferior iliac spine down to border of the iliac bones to the caudal edge of the sacrum and coccyx (C1–C2) as well as to the lateral sacral crest on a level with S3–S4 and posterior sacroiliac ligament on this line (Sashin, 1930; Gerlach and Lierse, 1992; Loukas et al., 2006). It inserts on the ischial tuberosity inferiorly (Gerlach and Lierse, 1992; Hammer et al., 2009; Bierry et al., 2014). As pelvic stabilizers (Hammer et al., 2019a), they are biomechanically significant as they help prevent the sacrum from tilting when shear forces are applied (Hatfield, 1971; Vleeming et al., 1989a; Vleeming et al., 1989b; van Wingerden et al., 1993; Woodley et al., 2005) by effectively counterbalancing nutation of the sacrum which firmly anchors the inferior sacrum to the ischium (Forst et al., 2006). These structures act to effectively compress and anchor the sacrum between the two ilia so that the irregular articular surfaces interlock together firmly providing 'force closure' the joint (Lee, 2007).

1.7   Vascular Anatomy

The common iliac and the internal iliac vessels lie directly anterior to the sacroiliac joints at the levels of L5-S2 with the superior gluteal vessels lying ventrally (slightly inferior) at S2 to S3 (Zoccali et al., 2015). The joint is supplied by branches from the anastomosis between the *median sacral artery* and the *lateral sacral branches of the internal iliac artery* which travel via the anterior sacral foramina and anastomose with the posterior sacral iliac blood supply from the superior and inferior gluteal arteries (Bernard and Cassidy, 1991). A nutrient artery of the ilium provides blood supply to the anterior sacroiliac joint region (Alla et al., 2013). It arises from the iliolumbar artery shown to arise variably from the common or the internal iliac artery to course across the sacroiliac joint to enter the nutrient foramen of the ilium (Figure 1.12) (Rusu et al., 2010).

Vascular branches arise from the inferior gluteal artery which travel close to the sacrospinous and sacrotuberous ligaments. These are shown to traverse the sacrotuberous ligament close to its sacral origin. This was found to occur via one artery in 69% of specimens and two arteries in 8% of specimens (Hammer et al., 2009). There is vast variation in both the origin and distribution of the blood supply to the sacrotuberous ligament. Vascular branches from the inferior and superior gluteal arteries enter the ligament close to the ischial tuberosity and sacrum in a variety of patterns (Figure 1.13). These can be in a combination of one to four

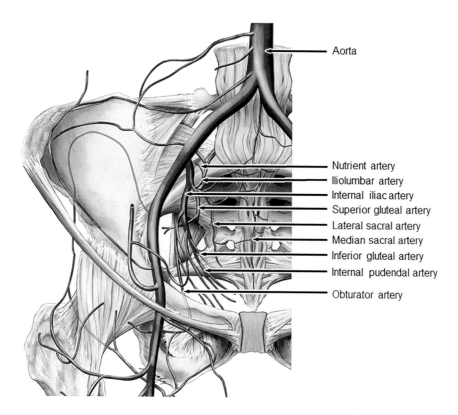

Aorta

Nutrient artery
Iliolumbar artery
Internal iliac artery
Superior gluteal artery
Lateral sacral artery
Median sacral artery
Inferior gluteal artery
Internal pudendal artery
Obturator artery

Figure 1.12 Arterial blood supply to the anterior region of the sacroiliac joint region (right side, anterior view).

branches of the inferior gluteal artery entering the sacrotuberous liga-ment with one to two branches of the superior gluteal artery (Lai et al., 2017). Abundance in blood supply is indicative of the proprioceptive func-tion of the sacrospinous-sacrotuberous ligament complex. Furthermore, the subchondral bone plate of the sacroiliac joint on both the iliac and sacral sides is penetrated by multiple blood vessels which are close to the articular cartilage (Kampen and Tillmann, 1998; Puhakka et al., 2004; Egund and Jurik, 2014).

The venous drainage of the joint occurs from tributary veins from the median and lateral sacral veins forming part of the anterior veinous drainage of the sacrum (Zeit and Cope, 1983; Bernard and Cassidy, 1991). The *Batson plexus* or 'vertebral venous plexus' found within the vertebrae and sacrum also contributes to the venous drainage (Figure 1.14), thereby forming a rich network of venous plexuses in the pelvic region (Groen et al., 1997; Nathoo et al., 2011).

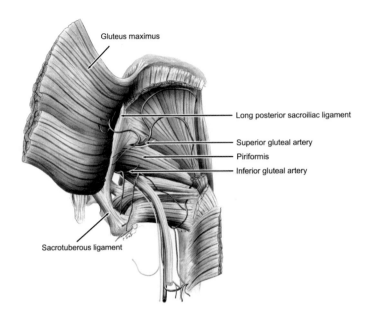

Figure 1.13 Blood supply of the posterior sacroiliac joint region (right side, posterior view).

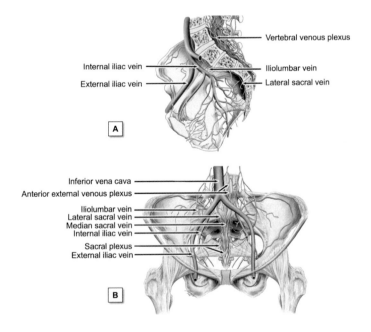

Figure 1.14 Venous drainage of pelvis and sacroiliac region: (A) Mediolateral view and (B) anterior view.

1.8 Innervation

The innervation of the sacroiliac joint is provided by the *segments L3 to S2 anteriorly* and *L4 to S4 posteriorly* (Poilliot et al., 2019b). Some studies report branches of superior gluteal nerves and the sacral plexus to contribute to the sacroiliac joint innervation. However, the innervation of the joint varies highly between individuals, as the pathways for innervation differ even between the same nerves.

The *anterior aspect* of the joint is mainly innervated by the *segments L4 to S2*, sometimes L3, and the sacral plexus or even the superior gluteal nerve (Figure 1.15) (Solonen, 1957; Ikeda, 1991; Grob et al., 1995; Diel et al., 2001; Cox et al., 2017). More specifically, the upper anterior portion of the sacroiliac joint is innervated by the ventral ramus of L5, and the lower portion by S2 or branches of the sacral plexus (Ikeda, 1991). Two studies found contributions of L4 and L5 (Szadek et al., 2008; Cox et al., 2017).

Further to this, the branches from the posterior lumbosacral rami (L5 to S3-S4) are the main innervation structures of the posterior aspect of the joint (Figure 1.16), and its neighboring structures (Ikeda, 1991; Grob et al.,

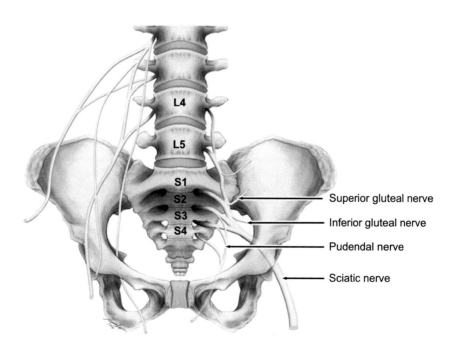

Figure 1.15 Innervation of the anterior sacroiliac region (anterior view).

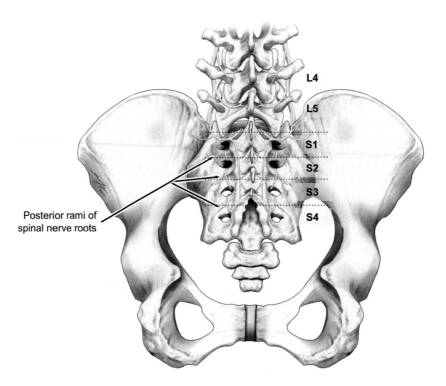

L4

L5

S1

S2

S3

S4

Posterior rami of
spinal nerve roots

Figure 1.16 Innervation of the posterior sacroiliac region (posterior view).

1995). This includes the interosseous, posterior and long posterior sacroiliac ligaments (Horwitz, 1939; Solonen, 1957; Bradley, 1974; Grob et al.,
1995; McGrath and Zhang, 2005), but also the sacrotuberous and sacrospinous ligaments (Fortin et al., 1999; Vilensky et al., 2002; Varga et al., 2008;
Mitchell and Vivian, 2011).

The dorsal lateral branches of S3 and S4 perforate the posterior sacroiliac ligaments, reach the skin via the gluteus medius muscle as medial
cluneal nerves and traverse downwards to reach the sacrotuberous ligament (Grob et al., 1995; McGrath and Zhang, 2005; McGrath et al., 2009).
The dorsal intermediate branches of the lumbar and sacral spinal nerves
likely also contribute to sacroiliac joint innervation, and are an area of
ongoing research (Kampsen, 2020; Tödtling, 2021).

Furthermore, the sacrotuberous ligament may receive supply from
the perforating ramus of the pudendal nerve (Hammer et al., 2009).
The lateral branches of the sacral dorsal rami arise from the sacral
foramina, radiating superiorly, laterally, or inferiorly across the dorsal
sacrum and travel through, superior or deep to the posterior sacroiliac
ligament (Mitchell and Vivian, 2011). Electrophysiological findings

from nerve fibers innervating the sacroiliac joint revealed that most were group III, high-threshold (Sakamoto et al., 2001). Furthermore, small fibers containing substance P and calcitonin gene-related polypeptide were found in the cartilage on either side and the surrounding ligaments (Szadek et al., 2010). These properties combined with fibers this size have been associated in the past with nociception in other parts and are most likely involved in the pain perception of the joint (Vleeming et al., 2012).

1.9 Myofascial Connections

The main compressors and stabilizers of the sacroiliac joint and lower spine are the muscles which directly influence force closure (Figure 1.17) (Vleeming et al., 1995a; Vleeming and Schuenke, 2019). It is said that muscles cross the sacroiliac joint but none directly impacts the joint (Grieve, 1976; Harrison et al., 1997; Foley and Buschbacher, 2006). However, this claim can be challenged as these muscles are involved in the force closure system, and therefore muscular imbalance will undoubtedly result in a

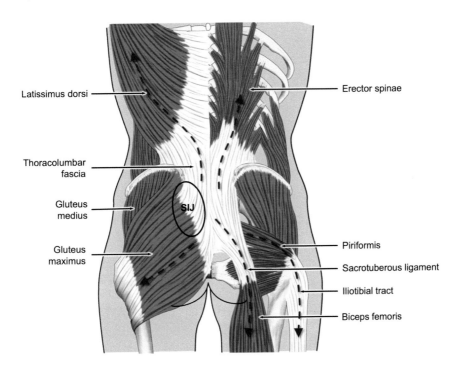

Figure 1.17 Posterior muscle system that form attachment sites to the sacroiliac joint (sacroiliac joint) region or sacroiliac joint ligaments. Blue arrows represent the tensions applied to the sacroiliac joint via the ligaments and muscles (posterior view). SIJ: sacroiliac joint.

biomechanical dysfunction. Muscles and fascia which may impact the sacroiliac joint (Cameron, 1907; Porterfield and DeRosa, 1990; Walker, 1992; Vleeming et al., 1995b; Oldreive, 1996; Harrison et al., 1997; Calvillo et al., 2000; Forst et al., 2006; Tuite, 2008; Robert et al., 2009; Hayashi et al., 2013) include:

- thoracolumbar fascia
- deep pelvic fascia
- latissimus dorsi muscle
- psoas major muscle
- quadratus lumborum muscle
- erector spinae
- lumbar multifidus muscles
- gluteus maximus muscle
- gluteus medius muscle
- coccygeus muscle
- piriformis muscle
- biceps femoris muscle
- semimembranosus muscle
- semitendinosus muscle
- transversus abdominis muscles

The *thoracolumbar fascia* can be regarded as a layered aponeurotic structure forming the retinaculum around the paraspinal muscles of the lower back and pelvic regions. As it envelops most of the postero-lateral part of the pelvic girdle, it provides attachment sites to various other muscular structures and provides stability to the lumbopelvic region, including the sacroiliac joint. The thoracolumbar fascia is composed of two distinct layers: an anterior and a posterior one. To provide stability to the lower back and the sacroiliac joint, both layers unite inferiorly to form a lumbar composite attachment to the posterior superior iliac spine and sacrotuberous ligament (Willard et al., 2012). It has other connections to the following muscles:

- erector spinae
- lumbar multifidus muscles
- gluteal muscles

The *deep pelvic fascia* has considerable attachment sites to structures around the sacroiliac joint. It attaches inferiorly along the course of the obturator internus muscle along the margin of the pubic arch and the sacrotuberous ligament. Posteriorly, the fascial and muscular margins attach to the greater sciatic notch and the base of the ischial spine. The obturator sheath is also present between the sacrospinous and sacrotuberous ligaments, ischial spine and the tendon of the obturator internus muscle (Cameron, 1907; Hammer et al., 2009). It has other connections to (Stecco et al., 2013):

- gluteus maximus muscle
- biceps femoris tendon

Literature has thoroughly commented on the fact that the *gluteus maximus* muscle attaches to the sacrotuberous and the long posterior sacroiliac ligament (Vleeming et al., 1989a; Vleeming et al., 1996; Woodley et al., 2005; Hammer et al., 2009; McGrath et al., 2009; Barker et al., 2014; Aldabe et al., 2019). On the posterior aspect, gluteus maximus arises from the superior lateral aspect to the inferior medial aspect as follows: the gluteus medius fascia (1), the ilium and thoracolumbar fascia (2), the erector spinae aponeurosis (3), the long posterior sacroiliac ligament (4), the sacral periosteum and sacrotuberous ligament (5) and finally the coccyx (6) For Amelie (Stecco et al., 2013; Barker et al., 2014) (Figure 1.18). It is also continuous with the fascia lata and iliotibial tract of the thigh (Stecco et al., 2013).

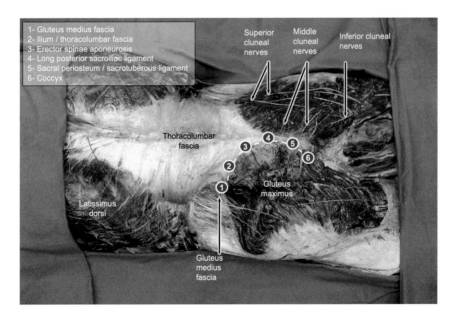

Figure 1.18 Superficial attachment sites of gluteus maximus on the posterior aspect. The hip bone attachments and the sacrotuberous ligament are not shown as deeper layers.

Source: Courtesy of Bettina Pretterklieber.

The *piriformis* muscle is often described as the only muscle having a direct attachment to the sacroiliac joint, crossing over the joint to pull the pelvis in an oblique direction (Alderink, 1991; Oldreive, 1996). The dorsal aspect of the piriformis muscle is continuous with the sacrotuberous ligament and the muscle fibers attach directly to the ventral part of the ligament (Vleeming et al., 1989a). However, the forces exerted by the piriformis muscle are relatively small when considering the lever across the joint and the muscle thickness. Furthermore, thick collagen fibers corresponding to the final sacrospinous were found in the postero-inferior margin of the coccygeus muscle (Hayashi et al., 2013).

The *erector spinae* muscles are composed of the iliocostalis, longissimus, and sacrospinalis muscles forming substructures with distinct functionality. Sacrospinalis has the most attachments to the sacroiliac area, which includes: the medial crest of the sacrum, the spinous processes of the lumbar vertebrae, and vertebral bodies T11 and T12. It also attaches to the posterior part of the inner lip of the iliac crests and the lateral sacral crests, blending with the sacrotuberous and posterior sacroiliac ligaments (Bogduk, 1980). In addition, the erector spinae muscles have fibers attaching to the dorsal aspect of the iliolumbar ligament and the medial fibers of the long posterior sacroiliac ligament (Vleeming et al., 1996; Pool-Goudzwaard et al., 2001; McGrath et al., 2009). These attachment tendons are sometimes confused with the various parts of the iliolumbar ligament such as in the case of Ashby et al. (2021) and Völker et al. (2021). What is described here is the quadratus lumborum epimysium arising from the dorsal aspect of L5 and fibers from the erector spinae from L4, whereas the iliolumbar ligament arises from the transverse process of L5 (Hammer et al., 2010; Poilliot et al., 2019b).

The *thoracolumbar transverso-spinal muscles*, which include the 'lumbar multifidus muscle', form a subgroup of paraspinal muscles which provide vertebral stability and a 'fine tuning' of spinal movements. They are located throughout the spine from the cervical part to the lumbar and sacral parts, including structures of the sacroiliac joint. The thoracolumbar transverso-spinal muscles are composed of various fleshy tendinous fascicles running caudo-laterally filling up the space on either side of the spinous processes of each vertebra (Cornwall et al., 2011). In the sacral region, the fascicles arise from the posterior sacrum as low as the sacral foramen of S4. They attach to the sacral tubercles of the intermediate crest, the median sacral crest, the erector spinae aponeurosis, the postero-medial surface of the posterior superior iliac spine and the medial aspect of the long posterior sacroiliac ligament (LPSL) (Bogduk, 1980; Cornwall et al., 2011). Caudally and medially, there is no fascia overlying the sacral tubercles and the thoracolumbar transverso-spinal muscles attach directly onto the sacral periosteum and multifidus muscle on the sacrum. They originate from L1 to L4 attaching inferiorly to the superior posterior superior iliac spine, sacroiliac joint region and sacral levels S2 and S3 on the medial sacrum (Cornwall et al., 2011). Fatty deposits are commonly observed within the erector spinae substructures (Pezolato et al., 2012). These deposits on one side may be indicative of degeneration (Parkkola et al., 1993).

On the other hand, adipocytes organized in compartments medially, provide a mechanical buffer zone for the perforating medial, intermediate, and lateral branches of the dorsal ramus of the spinal nerve (Saito et al., 2013).

The *biceps femoris* muscle has muscular attachments to the sacroiliac joint complex, in particular to the sacrotuberous ligament (Vleeming et al., 1989a; van Wingerden et al., 1993; Cornwall et al., 2011; Bierry et al., 2014; Aldabe et al., 2020). Van Wingerden et al. determined that the biceps femoris muscle attaches to the lower part of the superficial fibers of the sacrotuberous ligament, with some of its lateral deep fibers also connecting to the sacrotuberous ligament in some of the specimens (van Wingerden et al., 1993). Moreover, the biceps femoris muscle tendon connects to the sacrotuberous ligament with some having completely fused with the ligament (Vleeming et al., 1989a). Another study compared hamstring attachments in patients with pain and those with no pain. Results showed that the sacrotuberous ligament was continuous with the biceps femoris and the semitendinosus muscles in all of their specimens with no pain and in 88% of the patients with pain. The sacrotuberous ligament, however, was not continuous with the semimembranosus muscle in any of the cases (Bierry et al., 2014).

Finally, the iliolumbar ligament has various muscle attachments to muscles of the back and pelvis (Pool-Goudzwaard et al., 2001; Hammer et al., 2010), including:

- erector spinae muscles
- quadratus lumborum muscle
- iliacus muscle

In addition, the sacrotuberous ligament has attachments (Woodley et al., 2005; Aldabe et al., 2019) to the following muscles:

- the piriformis
- the obturator internus
- the semitendinosus
- the semimembranosus

1.10   *Joint Histology*

The features the sacroiliac joint presents histologically vary broadly from other joints. The joint has been described previously as a syndesmosis (Egund and Jurik, 2014), symphysis (Puhakka et al., 2004), amphiarthrosis (Gerlach and Lierse, 1992; Christ et al., 2001), diarthro-amphiarthrosis, or as a true diarthrodial joint with a synovial lining (Macdonald and Hunt, 1952; Bowen and Cassidy, 1981; Puhakka et al., 2004; Egund and Jurik, 2014) based on structural findings. These different interpretations may partly be due to interindividual variations in joint characteristics and to the age-related changes that the sacroiliac joint undergoes.

1.10.1   Bones of the Sacroiliac Joint

The subchondral bone lamellae below both the sacral and iliac auricular surfaces at the anterior sacroiliac joint region present high-density regions. In contrast, the posterior syndesmotic area is characterized to be discontinuous. Here, the bone lamellae are disrupted by ridges and groves, forming insertional points of the interosseous and posterior ligamentous apparatus. The sacral bone lamella remains unaltered over the course of aging, the iliac lamella undergoes thickening, likely as a consequence of the increasing shearing forces (Kampen and Tillmann, 1998). Bilaterally, the bone plates are penetrated by blood vessels (Kampen and Tillmann, 1998) and nerves (Szadek et al., 2010). Moreover, trabeculae emerging from the cancellous bone areas reinforce the subchondral bone plates, being more dominant on the sacral when compared to the iliac side.

1.10.2   Auricular Surface Cartilage

The auricular surfaces of the anterior sacroiliac joint area are covered bilaterally with cartilage (Fick, 1904; Egund and Jurik, 2014). On the sacral side, hyaline cartilage is found, which averages 0.5 to 2.1 mm in thickness (Kampen and Tillmann, 1998; Egund and Jurik, 2014). The cartilage on the iliac side first develops as fibrocartilage (Kampen and Tillmann, 1998; Egund and Jurik, 2014), and later transforms into hyaline cartilage (Kampen and Tillmann, 1998). Peripheral iliac areas remain fibrocartilaginous. Likewise, the auricular surface areas may fill with fibrocartilage as a consequence of ridge and groove formation (Puhakka et al., 2004). The iliac auricular cartilage is less thick when compared to the sacral side, averaging 0.7 to 1.2 mm (Kampen and Tillmann, 1998; Puhakka et al., 2004; Egund and Jurik, 2014). The iliac auricular cartilage has a relatively low glycosaminoglycan content (Kampen and Tillmann, 1998).

The proximal and distal third of the synovial joint are characterized by a poor to incomplete synovial lining (Puhakka et al., 2004; Egund and Jurik, 2014). The morphological changes of the cartilage include collagen demasking, chondrocyte clustering, irregularities and joint fissures that are seen at an early stage in life (Kampen and Tillmann, 1998). These changes are more pronounced on the iliac than on the sacral side (Kampen and Tillmann, 1998; Puhakka et al., 2004), begin in infancy, and become clearly visible in adolescents. However, these changes seem to be closely related to joint kinematics. Bipedal walking and upright posture seem to trigger events for the changes that the cartilage undergoes. Likely, the surface irregularities and roughness increase the frictional coefficient to enhanced the form closure, and therefore help minimize the energy expenditure for upright stance. Dense connections exist between the iliac cartilage and the surrounding ligaments (Figure 1.19) (Puhakka et al., 2004). Sometimes, the joint cavity is replaced by a proper fibrocartilaginous synchondrosis (Puhakka et al., 2004).

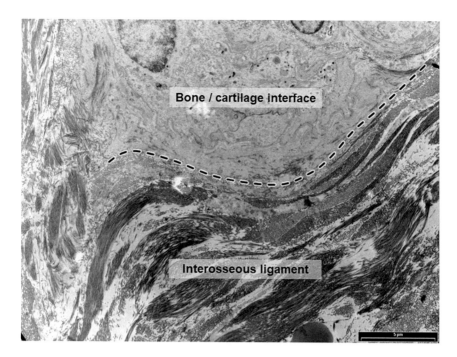

Figure 1.19 Scanning electron microscope of the transitional cartilage region between the articular and syndesmotic sacroiliac joint region.

1.10.3 Ligaments

Both the extrinsic and intrinsic ligaments of the sacroiliac joint are formed by large quantities of type 1 collagen. These collagens are aligned in large bundles along the directions of major force transmission. Between the sites of condensed ligaments, looser (reticular) areas are found. The characteristic features of the type 1 collagens in the sacroiliac joint ligaments can be seen microscopically (Figure 1.20A, C, D) and ultra-structurally (D periods or banding) (Figure 1.19). Failure of the ligaments is accompanied by hemorrhage, the loss of the collagen banding, loss of ligament orientation, and so-called collagen balls (Hammer et al., 2019b).

The *iliolumbar ligament* of an infant is formed by muscle fibers (Luk et al., 1986). Collagens begin to infiltrate the preformed ligament. This transformation is induced by the stresses caused by upright posture, and collagen infiltration extends from the most lateral aspect of the L5 costal process. Between the third and fifth life decades, the remaining muscle fibers vanish. At the age of 60, fatty infiltration is observed, combined with myxoid

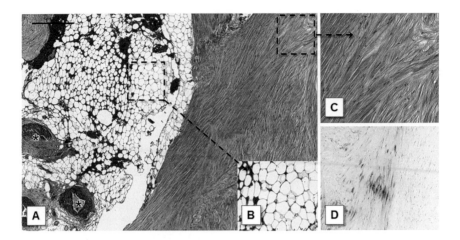

Figure 1.20 Hematoxylin- and eosin-stained slide of healthy sacroiliac joint ligaments and fat (A). Scale bar: 0.5 mm. Asterisks (*) are blood vessels. (B) Fat between the meshes of sacroiliac ligaments. (C) Close-up of the ligaments both running parallel and interwoven. (D) Giemsa stain of the ligamentous portion, with darker areas showing chondrification.

degeneration and calcification. The *sacrospinous* and *sacrotuberous ligaments* have a similar fate. Both ligaments originate from muscular origins. The sacrospinous ligament derives from the overlying coccygeus (posterior) muscle, remains densely connected and persists in having irregularly aligned muscle fibers within the ligament structure (Hayashi et al., 2013). The sacrotuberous ligament forms from a tendon attachment of the gluteus maximus muscle at the ischial tuberosity (Hayashi et al., 2013) and has the potential to ossify (Prescher and Bohndorf, 1993; Arora et al., 2009).

For the intrinsic sacroiliac joint ligaments, those fiber orientations seen on a macroscopic level continue to be seen microstructurally. Elastin can be found in the *anterior ligament*, while fenestrations may exist in both the fibrous (ligamentous) aspect and the synovial layer. The *interosseous and posterior ligaments* contain type 1 and 2 collagens, partial chondrification centers, and fat present between the fiber bundles at varying orientations (Figure 1.20B and D) (Poilliot et al., 2019a; Poilliot et al., 2020b). The fat seems to form pathways for the neurovascular pathways of the syndesmotic joint area (Fick, 1904; Puhakka et al., 2004). Such fenestrations are even visible with the naked eye for the long posterior ligaments.

1.10.4 Adipose Tissue

Fat is observed frequently within the sacroiliac joint ligaments. This is especially pronounced for the interosseous and posterior ligaments

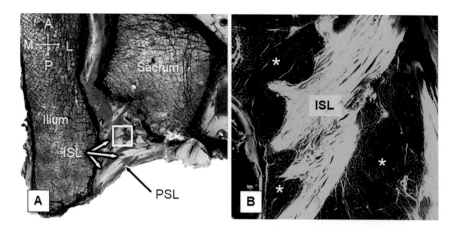

Figure 1.21 (A) Scan of an E-12 plastinated slice of a posterior sacroiliac joint region in the transverse plane. (B) Confocal laser microscopy images of the area represented with the white box on (A) at 10× magnification. The asterisks (*) represent the zones full of fat cells with black globular appearance between the meshes of interosseous sacroiliac ligament (ISL). A: anterior, L: lateral, M: medial, P: posterior, PSL: posterior sacroiliac ligament.

(Figure 1.21). Females have significantly higher amounts of fat in the central region of the syndesmotic complex. There is an age-dependent increase in fat in the inferior joint region in males, and an age-dependent decrease in the superior subregion in females (Poilliot et al., 2019a). Fat seems to provide a series of functions in the sacroiliac joint. First, it provides a pathway for the neurovascular structures to supply the syndesmotic part of the joint, especially the dorsal rami of the spinal nerves.

   Another yet neglected function is closely related to the collagen network of the ligaments encircling the adipocyte compartments formed by the fat in the posterior sacroiliac joint region. An analogue to this morphological relation between fat and ligaments is a mattress where the foam compares to the fat and the surrounding fabric compares to the ligament. Considering that fat is largely incompressible but deformable, compressive forces applied to the posterior pelvis cause the fat to deform. This deformation is limited by the distensibility of the ligament collagen network, typically averaging 15% (Hammer et al., 2013; Zwirner et al., 2019). As a consequence, fat serves as a damper in the posterior sacroiliac joint and mediates a function where the ligamentous structures become strained under tensile as well as compressive loading conditions (Figure 1.22). This finding is similar to the collagen septa forming the chambers of the plantar foot pad. Ligaments in the posterior joint may consequently be a functional adaptation rather than related to degeneration.

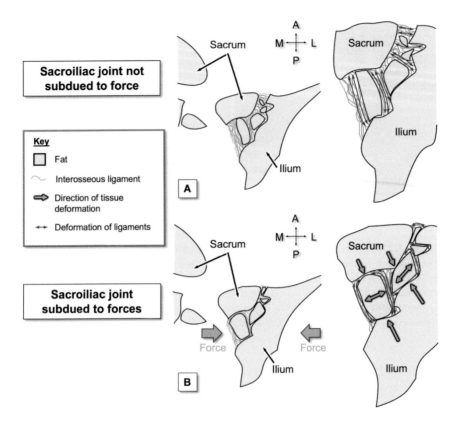

Figure 1.22 Schematic representation of fat in the posterior sacroiliac joint region. (A) The joint is under no force. Ligaments are tense and the fat is clearly visible between the interosseous ligamentous network. (B) The joint is subdued to force or load compressing the sacrum and ilium. The interosseous ligaments are no longer tense; the fat acts like a cushion between the ligamentous network. A: anterior, L: lateral, M: medial, P: posterior.

Source: Adapted from Hammer (2015).

1.10.5 Innervation of the Sacroiliac Joint Complex

The sacroiliac joint is densely innervated by lumbar and sacral spinal nerve branches. Ruffini endings, Pacinian corpuscles, and free nerve endings are found at the various parts of the joint and the attached ligaments, providing a broad range of slow- and fast-adapting mechanoreceptive afferents, accompanied by pain receptors. Denser fibers are found in the loose connective tissues of the sacroiliac joint, and, vice versa, beaded fibers are observed in the denser areas of the interosseous sacroiliac ligaments (Vilensky et al., 2002; Szadek et al., 2008). Pacinian corpuscles and free nerve endings are found in the interosseous ligaments (Vilensky et al., 2002; Szadek et al., 2008).

Pacinian, Ruffini, and free nerve endings are found in the iliolumbar ligament (Puhakka et al., 2004). Ruffini endings and ramifying terminals are found in the sacrospinous and sacrotuberous ligaments (Varga et al., 2008). Of interest, the cartilage and subchondral bone appear to be likewise densely innervated by free nerve endings (Szadek et al., 2010), an uncommon finding for healthy and intact joints.

References

Albee FH (1909) A study of the anatomy and the clinical importance of the sacroiliac joint. *Journal of the American Medical Association*, **LIII**, 1273–1276.

Aldabe D, Hammer N, Flack NAMS, Woodley SJ (2019) A systematic review of the morphology and function of the sacrotuberous ligament. *Clinical Anatomy*, **32**, 396–407.

Aldabe D, Milosavljevic S, Bussey MD (2020) A multivariate model for predicting PPGP considering postural adjustment parameters. *Musculoskeletal Science and Practice*, **48**, 102153.

Alderink G (1991) The sacroiliac joint: review of anatomy, mechanics, and function. *Journal of Orthopaedic and Sports Physical Therapy*, **13**, 71–84.

Alla SR, Roberts CS, Ojike NI (2013) Vascular risk reduction during anterior surgical approach sacroiliac joint plating. *Injury*, **44**, 175–177.

Anastasiou E, Chamberlain AT (2013) The sexual dimorphism of the sacro-iliac joint: an investigation using geometric morphometric techniques. *Journal of Forensic Sciences*, **58**, Suppl 1, S126–S134.

Arora J, Mehta V, Suri RK, Rath G (2009) Unilateral partial ossification of sacrotuberous ligament: anatomico-radiological evaluation and clinical implications. *Romanian Journal of Morphology and Embryology*, **50**, 505–508.

Ashby K, Yilmaz E, Mathkour M, et al. (2021) Ligaments stabilizing the sacrum and sacroiliac joint: a comprehensive review. *Neurosurgical Review*, **45**, 357–364.

Aulds MN (2019) Sacroiliac joint fusion in nulliparous and parous females and males. *American Journal of Physical Anthropology*, **168**, 10–10.

Bakland O, Hansen JH (1984) The "axial sacroiliac joint". *Anatomia Clinica*, **6**, 29–36.

Barker PJ, Hapuarachchi KS, Ross JA, Sambaiew E, Ranger TA, Briggs CA (2014) Anatomy and biomechanics of gluteus maximus and the thoracolumbar fascia at the sacroiliac joint. *Clinical Anatomy*, **27**, 234–240.

Basadonna PT, Gasparini D, Rucco V (1996) Iliolumbar ligament insertions: in vivo anatomic study. *Spine (Phila Pa 1976)*, **21**, 2313–2316.

Bellamy N, Park W, Rooney PJ (1983) What do we know about the sacroiliac joint? *Seminars in Arthritis and Rheumatism*, **12**, 282–313.

Benneman R (1979) Untersuchungen am Iliosakralgelenk des Menschen. *Verhandlungen der Anatomischen Gesellschaft*, **73**, 187–190.

Bernard TN, Cassidy JD (1991) The sacroiliac joint syndrome: pathophysiology, diagnosis and management. In *The Adult Spine: Principles and Practice* (ed Frymoyer JW), pp. 2107–2130. New York: Raven Press.

Bierry G, Simeone FJ, Borg-Stein JP, Clavert P, Palmer WE (2014) Sacrotuberous ligament: relationship to normal, torn, and retracted hamstring tendons on MR images. *Radiology*, **271**, 162–171.

Bogduk N (1980) A reappraisal of the anatomy of the human lumbar erector spinae. *Journal of Anatomy*, **131**, 525–540.

Bowen V, Cassidy JD (1981) Macroscopic and microscopic anatomy of the sacroiliac joint from embryonic life until the eighth decade. *Spine (Phila Pa 1976)*, **6**, 620–628.

Bradley KC (1974) The anatomy of backache. *ANZ Journal of Surgery*, **44**, 227–232.

Brooke R (1923) The sacro-iliac joint. *Journal of Anatomy*, **58**, 299–305.

Calvillo O, Skaribas I, Turnipseed J (2000) Anatomy and pathophysiology of the sacroiliac joint. *Current Review of Pain*, **4**, 356–361.

Cameron J (1907) The fascia of the pelvis. *Journal of Anatomy and Physiology*, **42**, 112–125.

Casaroli G, Bassani T, Brayda-Bruno M, Luca A, Galbusera F (2020) What do we know about the biomechanics of the sacroiliac joint and of sacropelvic fixation? A literature review. *Medical Engineering & Physics*, **76**, 1–12.

Christ B, Günther J, Frölich E, Huang R, Flöel H (2001) Morphological basis of Sell's irritation point of the sacroiliac joint. *Manuelle Medizin*, **39**, 241–245.

Cihan OF, Karabulut M, Kılınçoğlu V, Yavuz N (2020) The variations and degenerative changes of sacroiliac joints in asymptomatic adults. *Folia Morphologica (Warsz)*, **80**, 87–96.

Cornwall J, Stringer MD, Duxson M (2011) Functional morphology of the thoracolumbar transversospinal muscles. *Spine (Phila Pa 1976)*, **36**, E1053–E1061.

Cox M, Ng G, Mashriqi F, et al. (2017) Innervation of the anterior sacroiliac joint. *World Neurosurgery*, **107**, 750–752.

Cuppett M, Paladino J (2001) The anatomy and pathomechanics of the sacroiliac joint. *Athletic Therapy Today*, **6**, 6–14.

Dalstra M, Huiskes R (1995) Load transfer across the pelvic bone. *Journal of Biomechanics*, **28**, 715–724.

Demir M, Mavi A, Gumusburun E, Bayram M, Gursoy S, Nishio H (2007) Anatomical variations with joint space measurements on CT. *Kobe Journal of Medical Sciences*, **53**, 209–217.

Diel J, Ortiz O, Losada RA, Price DB, Hayt MW, Katz DS (2001) The sacrum: pathologic spectrum, multimodality imaging, and subspecialty approach. *Radiographics*, **21**, 83–104.

Dijkstra PF, Vleeming A, Stoeckart R (1989) Complex motion tomography of the sacroiliac joint—an anatomical and roentgenological study. *Fortschritte auf dem Gebiete der Röntgenstrahlen und der Nuklearmedizin*, **150**, 635–642.

Ebraheim N, Sabry FF, Nadim Y, Xu R, Yeasting RA (2000) Internal architecture of the sacrum in the elderly: an anatomic and radiographic study. *Spine (Phila Pa 1976)*, **25**, 292–297.

Egund N, Jurik AG (2014) Anatomy and histology of the sacroiliac joints. *Seminars in Musculoskeletal Radiology*, **18**, 332–339.

Ehara S, Elkhoury GY, Bergman RA (1988) The accessory sacroiliac joint—a common anatomic variant. *American Journal of Roentgenology*, **150**, 857–859.

Eichenseer PH, Sybert DR, Cotton JR (2011) A finite element analysis of sacroiliac joint ligaments in response to different loading conditions. *Spine*, **36**, E1446–E1452.

El Rafei M, Badr S, Lefebvre G, et al. (2018) Sacroiliac joints: anatomical variations on MR images. *European Radiology*, **28**, 5328–5337.

Fick R (1904) Anatomie der Gelenke. Kreuz-Darmbeingelenk. In *Handbuch der Anatomie und Mechanik der Gelenke unter Berücksichtigung der bewegenden Muskeln, vol. 2* (ed von Bardeleben K), pp. 289–303. Jena: Gustav Fischer.

Foley BS, Buschbacher RM (2006) Sacroiliac joint pain—anatomy, biomechanics, diagnosis, and treatment. *American Journal of Physical Medicine & Rehabilitation*, **85**, 997–1006.

Forst SL, Wheeler MT, Fortin JD, Vilensky JA (2006) The sacroiliac joint: anatomy, physiology and clinical significance. *Pain Physician*, **9**, 61–68.

Fortin JD, Kissling RO, O'Connor BL, Vilensky JA (1999) Sacroiliac joint innervation and pain. *American Journal of Orthopedics (Belle Mead NJ)*, **28**, 687–690.

Gerlach U, Lierse W (1992) Functional construction of the sacroiliac ligamentous apparatus. *Acta Anatomica*, **144**, 97–102.

Grieve GP (1976) The sacro iliac joint. *Physiotherapy*, **62**, 384–400.

Grob K, Neuhuber W, Kissling R (1995) Innervation of the human sacroiliacal joint. *Zeitschrift für Rheumatologie*, **54**, 117–122.

Groen RJ, Groenewegen HJ, van Alphen HA, Hoogland PV (1997) Morphology of the human internal vertebral venous plexus: a cadaver study after intravenous Araldite CY 221 injection. *Anatomical Record*, **249**, 285–294.

Hakim M (1937) Recherches sur l'articulation sacro-iliaque chez l'homme et les anthropoïdes. *Faculté de medecine de Paris*, **PhD**, Université de Paris.

Hammer N (2015) Morphologische und mechanische Untersuchungen zur Funktion des Beckenrings. *Medizinische Fakultät*, **Habilitation Thesis**, Universität Leipzig.

Hammer N, Höch A, Klima S, Le Joncour JB, Rouquette C, Ramezani M (2019a) Effects of cutting the sacrospinous and sacrotuberous ligaments. *Clinical Anatomy*, **32**, 231–237.

Hammer N, Ondruschka B, Fuchs V (2019b) Sacroiliac joint ligaments and sacroiliac pain: a case-control study on micro- and ultrastructural findings on morphologic alterations. *Pain Physician*, **22**, E615–E625.

Hammer N, Scholze M, Kibsgård T, et al. (2019c) Physiological in vitro sacroiliac joint motion: a study on three-dimensional posterior pelvic ring kinematics. *Journal of Anatomy*, **234**, 346–358.

Hammer N, Steinke H, Böhme J, Stadler J, Josten C, Spanel-Borowski K (2010) Description of the iliolumbar ligament for computer-assisted reconstruction. *Annals of Anatomy*, **192**, 162–167.

Hammer N, Steinke H, Lingslebe U, et al. (2013) Ligamentous influence in pelvic load distribution. *Spine Journal*, **13**, 1321–1330.

Hammer N, Steinke H, Slowik V, et al. (2009) The sacrotuberous and the sacrospinous ligament: a virtual reconstruction. *Annals of Anatomy*, **191**, 417–425.

Hanson P, Sonesson B (1994) The anatomy of the iliolumbar ligament. *Archives of Physical Medicine and Rehabilitation*, **75**, 1245–1246.

Harrison D, Harrison D, Troyanovich S (1997) The sacroiliac joint: a review of anatomy and biomechanics with clinical implications. *Journal of Manipulative and Physiological Therapeutics*, **20**, 607–617.

Hartford J, McCullen M, Harris R, Brown C (2000) The iliolumbar ligament: three-dimensional volume imaging and computer reformatting by magnetic resonance: a technical note. *Spine (Phila Pa 1976)*, **25**, 1098–1103.

Hatfield KD (1971) The preauricular sulcus. *Australasian Radiology*, **15**, 168–169.

Hayashi S, Kim JH, Rodríguez-Vázquez JF, et al. (2013) Influence of developing ligaments on the muscles in contact with them: a study of the annular ligament of the radius and the sacrospinous ligament in mid-term human fetuses. *Anatomy & Cell Biology*, **46**, 149–156.

Hoel RJ, Ledonio CG, Takahashi T, Polly DW, Jr. (2017) Sacral bone mineral density (BMD) assessment using opportunistic CT scans. *Journal of Orthopaedic Research*, **35**, 160–166.

Horwitz M (1939) The anatomy of (A) the lumbosacral nerve plexus—its relation to variations of vertebral segmentation, and (B), the posterior sacral nerve plexus. *Anatomical Record*, **74**, 91–107.

Ikeda R (1991) Innervation of the sacroiliac joint. Macroscopical and histological studies. *Nihon Ika Daigaku Zasshi*, **58**, 587–596.

İşcan MY, Derrick K (1984) Determination of sex from the sacroiliac joint: a visual assessment technique. *Florida Scientist*, **47**, 94–98.

Jesse MK, Kleck C, Williams A, et al. (2017) 3D morphometric analysis of normal sacroiliac joints: a new classification of surface shape variation and the potential implications in pain syndromes. *Pain Physician*, **20**, E701–E709.

Kampen WU, Tillmann B (1998) Age-related changes in the articular cartilage of human sacroiliac joint. *Anatomy and Embryology (Berl)*, **198**, 505–513.

Kampsen C (2020) Die dorsale SIG-innervation—Eine Grundlagenstudie. *Medizinische Fakultät, Institut für Anatomie I*, **MD Thesis**, Heinrich-Heine-Universität Düsseldorf.

Kiapour A, Joukar A, Elgafy H, Erbulut DU, Agarwal AK, Goel VK (2020) Biomechanics of the sacroiliac joint: anatomy, function, biomechanics, sexual dimorphism, and causes of pain. *International Journal of Spine Surgery*, **14**, 3–13.

Lai J, du Plessis M, Wooten C, et al. (2017) The blood supply to the sacrotuberous ligament. *Surgical and Radiologic Anatomy*, **39**, 953–959.

Lee D (2007) An integrated therapeutic approach to the treatment of the pelvic girdle. In *Movement, Stability and Lumbopelvic Pain: Integration and Research* (ed Vleeming A), pp. 621–638. Edinburgh: Churchill Livingstone.

Loukas M, Louis RG, Jr., Hallner B, Gupta AA, White D (2006) Anatomical and surgical considerations of the sacrotuberous ligament and its relevance in pudendal nerve entrapment syndrome. *Surgical and Radiologic Anatomy*, **28**, 163–169.

Luk KDK, Ho HC, Leong JCY (1986) The iliolumbar ligament—a study of its anatomy, development and clinical-significance. *Journal of Bone and Joint Surgery—British Volume*, **68**, 197–200.

Luschka H (1854) Die Kreuzdarmbeinfuge und die Schambeinfuge des Menschen. *Virchows Archiv für Pathologische Anatomie und Physiologie und für klinische Medicin*, **VII**, 299–316.

Macdonald GR, Hunt TE (1952) Sacroiliac joints; observations on the gross and histological changes in the various age groups. *Canadian Medical Association Journal*, **66**, 157–163.

McGrath MC, Nicholson H, Hurst P (2009) The long posterior sacroiliac ligament: a histological study of morphological relations in the posterior sacroiliac region. *Joint Bone Spine*, **76**, 57–62.

McGrath MC, Zhang M (2005) Lateral branches of dorsal sacral nerve plexus and the long posterior sacroiliac ligament. *Surgical and Radiologic Anatomy*, **27**, 327–330.

McLauchlan GJ, Gardner DL (2002) Sacral and iliac articular cartilage thickness and cellularity: relationship to subchondral bone end-plate thickness and cancellous bone density. *Rheumatology (Oxford)*, **41**, 375–380.

Mitchell B, Vivian D (2011) Sacroiliac joint pain: procedures for diagnosis and treatment. In *Pain Procedures in Clinical Practice*, pp. 391–405. Philadelphia: Elsevier.

Nathoo N, Caris EC, Wiener JA, Mendel E (2011) History of the vertebral venous plexus and the significant contributions of Breschet and Batson. *Neurosurgery*, **69**, 1007–1014.

Okumura M, Ishikawa A, Aoyama T, et al. (2017) Cartilage formation in the pelvic skeleton during the embryonic and early-fetal period. *PLoS ONE*, **12**, e0173852.

Oldreive WL (1996) A critical review of the literature on the anatomy and biomechanics of the sacroiliac joint. *Journal of Manual and Manipulative Therapy*, **4**, 157–165.

Ou-Yang DC, York PJ, Kleck CJ, Patel VV (2017) Diagnosis and management of sacroiliac joint dysfunction. *Journal of Bone and Joint Surgery—American Volume*, **99**, 2027–2036.

Paquin JD, Vanderrest M, Marie PJ, et al. (1983) Biochemical and morphologic studies of cartilage from the adult human sacroiliac joint. *Arthritis and Rheumatism*, **26**, 887–895.

Parkkola R, Rytokoski U, Kormano M (1993) Magnetic resonance imaging of the discs and trunk muscles in patients with chronic low back pain and healthy control subjects. *Spine (Phila Pa 1976)*, **18**, 830–836.

Peretz AM, Hipp JA, Heggeness MH (1998) The internal bony architecture of the sacrum. *Spine (Phila Pa 1976)*, **23**, 971–974.

Petersen O (1905) Über Artikulationsflächen an der Unterfläche des Os sacrum. *Anatomischer Anzeiger*, **26**, 521–524.

Pezolato A, de Vasconcelos EE, Defino HL, Nogueira-Barbosa MH (2012) Fat infiltration in the lumbar multifidus and erector spinae muscles in subjects with sway-back posture. *European Spine Journal*, **21**, 2158–2164.

Poilliot A, Doyle T, Tomlinson J, Zhang M, Zwirner J, Hammer N (2019a) Quantification of fat in the posterior sacroiliac joint region: fat volume is sex and age dependant. *Scientific Reports*, **9**, 14935.

Poilliot A, Doyle T, Kurosawa D, et al. (2021) Computed tomography osteoabsorptiometry-based investigation on subchondral bone plate alterations in sacroiliac joint dysfunction. *Scientific Reports*, **11**, 8652.

Poilliot A, Doyle T, Tomlinson J, Zhang M, Zwirner J, Hammer N (2019a) Quantification of fat in the posterior sacroiliac joint region: fat volume is sex and age dependant. *Scientific Reports*, **9**, 14935.

Poilliot A, Li KC, Müller-Gerbl M, et al. (2020a) Subchondral bone strength of the sacroiliac joint a combined approach using computed tomography osteoabsorptiometry (CT-OAM) imaging and biomechanical validation. *Journal of Mechanical Behavior of Biomedical Materials*, **111**, 103978.

Poilliot A, Tannock M, Zhang M, Zwirner J, Hammer N (2020b) Quantification of fat in the posterior sacroiliac joint region applying a semi-automated segmentation method. *Computer Methods and Programs in Biomedicine*, **191**, 105386.

Poilliot A, Zwirner J, Doyle T, Hammer N (2019b) A systematic review of the normal sacroiliac joint anatomy and adjacent tissues for pain physicians. *Pain Physician*, **22**, E247–E274.

Pool-Goudzwaard AL, Kleinrensink GJ, Snijders CJ, Entius C, Stoeckart R (2001) The sacroiliac part of the iliolumbar ligament. *Journal of Anatomy*, **199**, 457–463.

Porterfield J, DeRosa C (1990) The sacroiliac joint. In *Orthopaedic and Sports Physical Therapy* (ed Gould JA), pp. 553–573. St. Louis: C.V. Mosby Company.

Postacchini R, Trasimeni G, Ripani F, Sessa P, Perotti S, Postacchini F (2017) Morphometric anatomical and CT study of the human adult sacroiliac region. *Surgical and Radiologic Anatomy*, **39**, 85–94.

Prassopoulos PK, Faflia CP, Voloudaki AE, Gourtsoyiannis NC (1999) Sacroiliac joints: anatomical variants on CT. *Journal of Computer Assisted Tomography*, **23**, 323–327.

Prescher A, Bohndorf K (1993) Anatomical and radiological observations concerning ossification of the sacrotuberous ligament: is there a relation to spinal diffuse idiopathic skeletal hyperostosis (DISH)? *Skeletal Radiology*, **22**, 581–585.

Puhakka KB, Melsen F, Jurik AG, Boel LW, Vesterby A, Egund N (2004) MR imaging of the normal sacroiliac joint with correlation to histology. *Skeletal Radiology*, **33**, 15–28.

Rana SH, Farjoodi P, Haloman S, et al. (2015) Anatomic evaluation of the sacroiliac joint: a radiographic study with implications for procedures. *Pain Physician*, **18**, 583–592.

Resnick D, Niwayama G, Goergen TG (1975) Degenerative disease of the sacroiliac joint. *Investigative Radiology*, **10**, 608–621.

Robert R, Salaud C, Hamel O, Hamel A, Philippeau JM (2009) Anatomie des douleurs de l'articulation sacro-iliaque. *Revue Du Rhumatisme*, **76**, 727–733.

Rosatelli A, Agur A, Chhaya S (2006) Anatomy of the interosseous region of the sacroiliac joint. *Journal of Orthopaedic and Sports Physical Therapy*, **36**, 200–208.

Rucco V, Basadonna PT, Gasparini D (1996) Anatomy of the iliolumbar ligament: a review of its anatomy and a magnetic resonance study. *American Journal of Physical Medicine & Rehabilitation*, **75**, 451–455.

Rusu MC, Cergan R, Dermengiu D, et al. (2010) The iliolumbar artery—anatomic considerations and details on the common iliac artery trifurcation. *Clinical Anatomy*, **23**, 93–100.

Saito T, Steinke H, Miyaki T, et al. (2013) Analysis of the posterior ramus of the lumbar spinal nerve: the structure of the posterior ramus of the spinal nerve. *Anesthesiology*, **118**, 88–94.

Sakamoto N, Yamashita T, Takebayashi T, Sekine M, Ishii S (2001) An electrophysiologic study of mechanoreceptors in the sacroiliac joint and adjacent tissues. *Spine*, **26**, E468–471.

Sashin D (1930) A critical analysis or the anatomy and the pathologic changes of the sacro-iliac joints. *Journal of Bone and Joint Surgery*, **12**, 891–910.

Schunke B, Bernard G (1938) The anatomy and development of the sacro-iliac joint in man. *Anatomical Record*, **72**, 313–331.

Seligman S (1935) Articulatio sacro-iliaca accessoria. *Anatomischer Anzeiger Bd*, **79**, 225–241.

Simkin P, Graney D, Fiechtner J (1980) Roman arches, human joints, and disease: differences between convex and concave sides of joints. *Arthritis & Rheumatology*, **23**, 1308–1311.

Snijders CJ, Vleeming A, Stoeckart R (1993) Transfer of lumbosacral load to iliac bones and legs. Part 1: biomechanics of self-bracing of the sacroiliac joints and its significance for treatment and exercise. *Clinical Biomechanics*, **8**, 285–294.

Solonen KA (1957) The sacroiliac joint in the light of anatomical, roentgenological and clinical studies. *Acta Orthopaedica Scandinavica, Supplement*, **27**, 1–127.

Stecco A, Gilliar W, Hill R, Fullerton B, Stecco C (2013) The anatomical and functional relation between gluteus maximus and fascia lata. *Journal of Bodywork and Movement Therapies*, **17**, 512–517.

Steinke H, Hammer N, Lingslebe U, Höch A, Klink T, Böhme J (2014) Ligament-induced sacral fractures of the pelvis are possible. *Clinical Anatomy*, **27**, 770–777.

Steinke H, Hammer N, Slowik V, et al. (2010) Novel insights into the sacroiliac joint ligaments. *Spine (Phila Pa 1976)*, **35**, 257–263.

Szadek KM, Hoogland PVJM, Zuurmond WWA, de Lange JJ, Perez RSGM (2008) Nociceptive nerve fibers in the sacroiliac joint in humans. *Regional Anesthesia and Pain Medicine*, **33**, 36–43.

Szadek KM, Hoogland PVJM, Zuurmond WWA, De Lange JJ, Perez RSGM (2010) Possible nociceptive structures in the sacroiliac joint cartilage: an immunohistochemical study. *Clinical Anatomy*, **23**, 192–198.

Szadek KM, van der Wurff P, van Tulder MW, Zuurmond WW, Perez RS (2009) Diagnostic validity of criteria for sacroiliac joint pain: a systematic review. *Journal of Pain*, **10**, 354–368.

Tague RG, Lovejoy CO (1986) The obstetric pelvis of A.L. 288–1 (Lucy). *Journal of Human Evolution*, **15**, 237–255.

Tödtling M (2021) Verlauf der Rami dorsales inklusive Differenzierung der Rami laterales et mediales innerhalb der autochthonen Rückenmuskulatur mit besonderer Berücksichtigung des minimalinvasiven dorsalen Zuganges zur Wirbelsäule. *Abteilung für Anatomie*, **MD thesis**, Medizinische Universität Wien.

Tok Umay S, Korkmaz M (2020) Frequency of anatomical variation of the sacroiliac joint in asymptomatic young adults and its relationship with sacroiliac joint degeneration. *Clinical Anatomy*, **33**, 839–843.

Trevathan W (1987) *Human Birth: An Evolutionary Perspective*. New Brunswick, NJ: Transaction Publishers.

Trotter M (1940) A common anatomical variation in the sacro-iliac region. *Journal of Bone and Joint Surgery*, **22**, 293–299.

Tuite M (2008) Sacroiliac joint imaging. *Seminars in Musculoskeletal Radiology*, **12**, 72–82.

Uhthoff HK (1993) Prenatal development of the iliolumbar ligament. *Journal of Bone and Joint Surgery. British*, **75**, 93–95.

Valojerdy MR, Hogg DA (1990) Anatomical note: the occurrence of accessory sacroiliac joints in man. *Clinical Anatomy*, **3**, 257–260.

van Wingerden JP, Vleeming A, Snijders CJ, Stoeckart R (1993) A functional-anatomical approach to the spine-pelvis mechanism: interaction between the biceps femoris muscle and the sacrotuberous ligament. *European Spine Journal*, **2**, 140–144.

Varga E, Dudas B, Tile M (2008) Putative proprioceptive function of the pelvic ligaments: biomechanical and histological studies. *Injury—International Journal of the Care of the Injured*, **39**, 858–864.

Vilensky JA, O'Connor BL, Fortin JD, et al. (2002) Histologic analysis of neural elements in the human sacroiliac joint. *Spine*, **27**, 1202–1207.

Vleeming A, Mooney V, Dorman T, Snijders C, Stoeckart R (1997) *Movement, Stability, and Low Back Pain: The Essential Role of the Pelvis*. New York: Churchill Livingstone.

Vleeming A, Pool-Goudzwaard AL, Hammudoghlu D, Stoeckart R, Snijders C, Mens J (1996) The function of the long dorsal sacroiliac ligament: its implication for understanding low back pain. *Spine (Phila Pa 1976)*, **21**, 556–562.

Vleeming A, Pool-Goudzwaard AL, Stoeckart R, Van Wingerden JP, Snijders CJ (1995a) The posterior layer of the thoracolumbar fascia—its function in load-transfer from spine to legs. *Spine (Phila Pa 1976)*, **20**, 753–758.

Vleeming A, Schuenke M (2019) Form and force closure of the sacroiliac joints. *Physical Medicine and Rehabilitation*, **11**, S24–S31.

Vleeming A, Schuenke M, Masi A, Carreiro J, Danneels L, Willard F (2012) The sacroiliac joint: an overview of its anatomy, function and potential clinical implications. *Journal of Anatomy*, **221**, 537–567.

Vleeming A, Snijders C, Stoeckart R, Mens J (1995b) A new light on low back pain. In *Interdisciplinary World Congress on Low Back Pain the Integrated Function of the Lumbar Spine and Sacroiliac Joints* (eds Vleeming A, Mooney V, Snijders C, Dorman T), pp. 9–11. San Diego: University of California.

Vleeming A, Stoekart R, Snijders C (1989a) The sacrotuberous ligament: a conceptual approach to its dynamic role in stabilizing the sacroiliac joint. *Clinical Biomechanics*, **4**, 201–203.

Vleeming A, Van Wingerden J, Snijders C, Stoeckart R, Stijnen T (1989b) Load application to the sacrotuberous ligament; influences on sacroiliac joint mechanics. *Clinical Biomechanics*, **4**, 204–209.

Völker A, Steinke H, Heyde CE (2021) The sacroiliac joint as a cause of pain—review of the sacroiliac joint morphology and models for pain genesis. *Zeitschrift für Orthopädie und Unfallchirurgie*. doi: 10.1055/a-1398-6055. Epub ahead of print.

Waldrop JT, Ebraheim NA, Yeasting RA, Jackson WT (1993) The location of the sacroiliac joint on the outer table of the posterior ilium. *Journal of Orthopaedic Trauma*, **7**, 510–513.

Walker J (1992) The sacroiliac joint: a critical review. *Physical Therapy*, **72**, 903–916.

Weisl H (1954) The ligaments of the sacroiliac joint examined with particular reference to their function. *Acta Anatomica*, **20**, 201–213.

Willard FH, Vleeming A, Schuenke MD, Danneels L, Schleip R (2012) The thoracolumbar fascia: anatomy, function and clinical considerations. *Journal of Anatomy*, **221**, 507–536.

Woodley S, Kennedy E, Mercer S (2005) Anatomy in practice: the sacrotuberous ligament. *New Zealand Journal of Physiotherapy*, **33**, 91–94.

Zeit RM, Cope C (1983) Anatomy of the sacral venous plexus. *AJR American Journal of Roentgenology*, **140**, 143–144.

Zoccali C, Skoch J, Patel AS, Walter CM, Maykowski P, Baaj AA (2015) The surgical neurovascular anatomy relating to partial and complete sacral and sacroiliac resections: a cadaveric, anatomic study. *European Spine Journal*, **24**, 1109–1113.

Zoccali C, Skoch J, Patel AS, et al. (2016) The surgical anatomy of the lumbosacroiliac triangle: a cadaveric study. *World Neurosurgery*, **88**, 36–40.

Zwirner J, Babian C, Ondruschka B, et al. (2019) Tensile properties of the human iliotibial tract depend on height and weight. *Medical Engineering & Physics*, **69**, 85–91.

chapter two

Biomechanics of the Sacroiliac Joint

Niels Hammer and Amélie Poilliot

Contents

The sacroiliac joint is designed to provide elasticity and load-induced deformation to a certain, well-defined extent. Though the movements observed both clinically and experimentally are minute, the existence of all morphological features of a (synovial) joint underline the importance the sacroiliac joint has as a load distribution zone of the osseous pelvis (horizontally) and of the lumbosacral transition with the lower extremities. The function of the sacroiliac joint is two fold: a movement-mediating and a shock-absorbing function. To understand how both these functions can be combined to be a morphological unit, it is important to expand the concept on sacroiliac joint kinematics beyond the joint itself but to the lumbar spine. This includes the lumbosacral junction, the hip joint, and the pubic symphysis in the scope of kinematic chains. This concept helps explain the movement-mediating kinematic function to compensate for movements induced via the lumbar spine and (anterior) pelvic ring. The shock-absorbing function of the sacroiliac joint lessens peak forces applied to the pelvic girdle and distributes them to the respective contralateral side of the pelvis and both lower limbs (Dontigny, 1985; Toyohara et al., 2020). This stress-relieving action would be ineffective if the pelvis formed a solid ring, as bone elasticity would fail, dissipating a sufficient quantity of energy if the pelvis was loaded suddenly

DOI: 10.1201/9781003348160-2

and extensively. In consequence, if the pelvis was a solid bone, both the adjacent spine and hip region would be damage-prone from the various bipedal functions (Vleeming et al., 2012; Toyohara et al., 2020).

2.1   Normal Sacroiliac Kinematics— Rotation, Translation, Nutation, and Integration in Two Leg Stance

Movement at the joint is limited, rotation arguably to a maximum of 1–3° or less in all three planes, and the articulating bones and sacroiliac ligaments reduce the possible extent of gliding rotary movement (Snijders et al., 1993; Slipman et al., 2001; Buford et al., 2010; Malarvizhi et al., 2017; Hammer et al., 2019c). Because of the ridges and grooves existing at the cartilaginous auricular joint surface, a higher coefficient of friction exists for the sacroiliac joint when compared to other joints (Bernard and Cassidy, 1991; Kampen and Tillmann, 1998; Puhakka et al., 2004). Increased friction helps minimize joint movements under physiologic loading. Additionally, the energy expenditure of the surrounding muscles, required to create a positional equilibrium of the joint, partners in an upright body posture. Under the conditions of body weight loading, rotations and translations of the sacroiliac joint are within the sub-millimeter and sub-degree range (Hammer and Klima, 2019; Hammer et al., 2019c). The fat present in the interosseous and posterior sacroiliac joints seems to be relevant to diminish load peaks, and to translate all loads exerted to the joint in ligament strain irrespective of the direction of the force vector (Poilliot et al., 2019). Recent numerical investigations provide first evidence in favor of this theory (Ramezani et al., 2019). It was shown here that the orientations of the interosseous and (short) posterior ligaments had less influence in pelvis deformation than initially thought (Ramezani et al., 2019).

The minimal but observable sacroiliac joint mobility provides sufficient flexibility to facilitate the intra-pelvic load transfer and also to and from the spine to the lower extremities (Lee, 2007). Anatomically, the sacrum is 'suspended' between the ilia by the meshes of ligaments surrounding the joint at varying directions (Dontigny, 1985). When standing upright on both legs, the weight of the body transmits forces ranging between 300 N to 1750 N (30 to 175 kg) through the lumbar vertebrae to the sacrum (Dontigny, 1985; Miller et al., 1987; Bernard and Cassidy, 1991; Hammer et al., 2019c). Much larger forces may occur under dynamic or unphysiological events, for example in case of trauma to the posterior pelvis. As these forces occur anterior to the axis of the loaded sacroiliac joint, the superior sacrum region is depressed anterior-inferiorly around a moving center axis of rotation in a 'tram-rail' type of motion, with the combined movement pattern termed *nutation* (Figure 2.1) (McGregor and

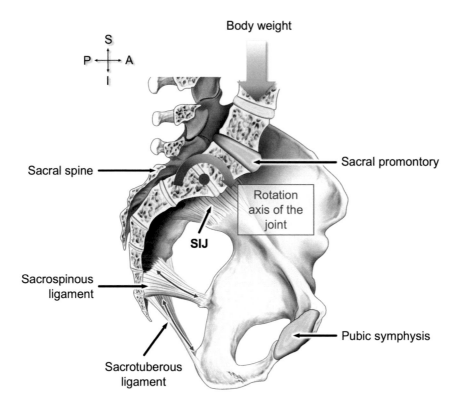

Figure 2.1 Nutation of the sacroiliac joint under axial loading (mediolateral view). A: anterior, I: inferior, P: posterior, S: superior, SIJ: sacroiliac joint.

Cassidy, 1983). In consequence, the inferior translation of the sacrum relative to both ilia tightens the posterior sacroiliac joint ligaments, resulting in an inwards rotation of the iliac wings to the sacrum in a sagittal axis (Figure 2.2), drawing the ilia and sacrum firmly together.

The sacroiliac joint complex consequently interlocks in a compressive manner as a consequence of axial loading, facilitated by the two phenomena called 'force closure' and 'form closure'. The first is achieved via the muscular system and the latter via the ligaments and bony structure of the auricular surfaces (Figure 2.3) (Dontigny, 1985; Snijders et al., 1993; Jordan, 2006; Vleeming et al., 2012; Booth and Morris, 2019; Zlomislic and Garfin, 2019), though both are interlinked inseparably. There is no term on the combined movement of nutation at the (anterior cartilaginous) sacroiliac joint and the rotations of the iliac wings yet. We suggest naming this movement *sacroiliac integration*, appreciating the complex, multidimensional movement of the joint elements (Figure 2.2).

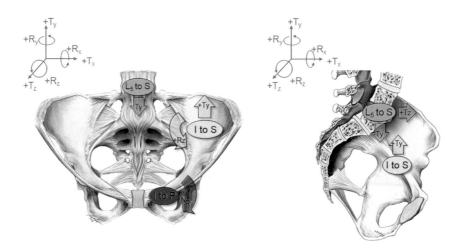

Figure 2.2 Schematic representation of the kinematics of the so-called sacroiliac integration of the pelvic girdle, each bone (L5, sacrum, ilium) to one another. Left depicts an anterior view, right a mediolateral view. Straight arrows represent translation (T) movements; rounded arrows represent a rotational (R) movement. I: ilium, L_5: fifth lumbar vertebra, P: pubic symphysis, S: sacrum.

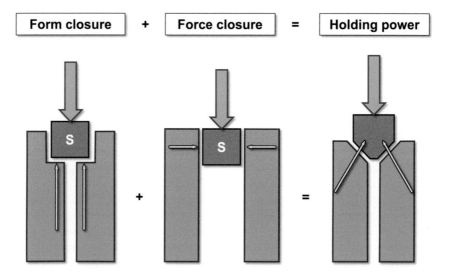

Figure 2.3 Schematic diagram of form and force closure. Blue arrow is the force transferred to the pelvic girdle. Yellow arrows represent the forces applied to the sacroiliac joints which actively compress the sacrum (S) between the ilia via the ligaments and bony structures during form closure and the muscles during force closure.

Nutation pre-strains the ligamentous structures maintaining the integrity of the joint, which effectively prepare it for an increase in load. This slight freedom of movement of the inferior sacrum in relation to the hip bones provides flexibility to the sacroiliac region when the vertebral column endures an increase in load and when lumbosacral flexion and extension occur (Forst et al., 2006; Zlomislic and Garfin, 2019). The relative flatness of the auricular surfaces of the sacroiliac joint allows it to withstand high compression and torsional motion; however, this configuration is unsuitable for forces acting transversely, thereby making the joint vulnerable to shear forces (Snijders et al., 1993; Kiapour et al., 2020). Rotation is counterbalanced by the sacrospinous and sacrotuberous ligaments, which anchor the inferior sacrum to the ischium (Forst et al., 2006), while counterrotation is counterbalanced by the long posterior sacroiliac ligaments (Eichenseer et al., 2011; Kiapour et al., 2020). Inferior translation is minimized by the interosseous and short posterior sacroiliac as well as the iliolumbar ligaments, while the long posterior sacroiliac, sacrospinous, and sacrotuberous ligaments minimize superior translation. These ligaments are closely connected to the erector spinae and quadratus lumborum, the gluteal muscles, the pelvic muscles (coccygeus, internal obturator, piriformis), and the hamstrings.

The erector spinae, psoas major, and gluteus maximus muscles load and extend the spine and pelvis. The erector spinae induces sacroiliac joint nutation which, as a result, tenses the interosseous, sacrotuberous, and sacrospinous ligaments (Vleeming et al., 2012). They act to principally pull the iliac bones together, constraining nutation mostly on the cranial side, whereas the caudal aspect tends to gape (Snijders et al., 1993; Vleeming et al., 2012). Furthermore, the latissimus dorsi muscle via the thoracolumbar fascia, piriformis, and gluteus maximus muscle can force the sacroiliac joints together because of the multiple attachment points of these muscles to the surrounding ligamentous structures (Forst et al., 2006; Enix and Mayer, 2019). Contraction of the transverse abdominis muscle has also been shown to decrease the laxity of the joint, suggesting that a strong core is beneficial for sacroiliac biomechanical function (Schmidt et al., 2018; Dontigny, 1979; Richardson et al., 2002). The pelvis works as a kinematic chain jointly with the lumbosacral junction and sacroiliac joints posteriorly and the pubic symphysis anteriorly. Under physiological loading conditions, L5 is transposed anterior-inferiorly relative to the sacrum (Hammer et al., 2019c). Additionally, small anterior rotations occur at the pubic symphysis anchoring both pubic bones together (Walheim and Selvik, 1984; Hammer et al., 2019c).

Beyond the movements observed within the sacroiliac joint, the adjacent segments seem to play an equally important role in pelvic ring kinematics. With loads being applied via the lumbar spine, the lumbosacral transition deforms markedly more than the sacroiliac joint (Hammer et al., 2019c). This motion is primarily an extension (Figure 2.2). Equally, the pubic symphysis plays a role in load dissipation. It not only connects both sacroiliac joints via the innominate bones anteriorly, but also compensates for differing loading directions between both sacroiliac joints, for example, in single leg stance or when walking. Compressive, tensile, and shear forces are observed at the pubic symphysis as a result (Figure 2.4), which is morphologically reflected in the presence of hyaline and fibrocartilage as well as dense ligaments. Two other important yet so far neglected segments in this chain of motion are the innominate bones themselves. At first glance the innominate bones seem to be rigid structures, contributing little to load dissipation. However, the extremely long lever arms of the innominate bones, totaling more than 150 millimeters, account for significant displacement with large interindividual variation as a consequence of load application (Solomon et al., 2014). As a result, a small but observable deformation can be found within the ilia when loaded, indicative of innominate bone elasticity.

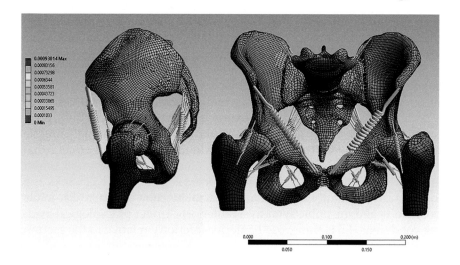

Figure 2.4 Virtual reconstruction of the osteo-ligamentous pelvis showing deformations under physiologic loading in two leg stance. Peak deformations are observed at the lumbosacral transition. Color code is used to visualize areas of large deformation (red) and areas of minute deformation (blue). Left depicts the lateromedial view, right the anterior view.

2.2   Altered Loading Patterns in Single Leg Stance and When Walking

When compared to the static situation of bilateral stance, single leg stance and walking induce markedly altered loading patterns at the sacroiliac joint. These changes in joint loading are not only due to increased loading on the side with the leg in the (ground) contact phase or the lift phase of the other side (Toyohara et al., 2020). The muscles allowing for this posture add stresses to the sacroiliac joints on both sides. Further to this, walking induces further the accelerations and decelerations to both sacroiliac joints as connective segments between the lower limbs and the trunk (Toyohara et al., 2020).

In single leg stance, the sacroiliac joint on the side with ground contact shows the typical signs of nutation, with a forward rotation of the sacral promontory and an inferior rotation of the sacrum relative to the ipsilateral ilium. The inward rotation of the ilium to the sacrum is diminished by the inferior portion of the gluteus maximus muscle and the gluteus medius, minimus, and the tensor fasciae latae due to their insertions lateral or inferior to the axis of this movement. In consequence, the contact forces of the sacroiliac joint on the standing side are increased and shifted inferiorly. Moreover, the erector spinae and lumbar multifidi, quadratus lumborum and psoas major muscles increase the shear forces at the sacroiliac joint, as it creates an abutment jointly with the hip joint of the standing side. The sacroiliac joint on the unloaded side yields a more typical counter nutation movement, where joint contact forces are lowered and shifted superiorly.

The walking condition exerts vastly changing force vectors to both sacroiliac joints. Similar to the standing position, the sacroiliac joint of the side in the stance phase shows the typical nutation pattern, while the joint on the side in the swing phase shows a counternutation pattern (Toyohara et al., 2020). Given the dynamic nature of walking, peak stresses at the auricular joint surfaces and sacroiliac ligaments are more extensive and shorter in duration when compared to the static standing position. The distortion the pelvis undergoes in this dynamic situation is mainly attributed to the sacroiliac joints. One of the key muscles of clinical relevance in the dynamic setting seems to be the rectus femoris. Though it does not directly move the sacroiliac joint, its insertion to the anterior inferior iliac spine exerts a long lever arm, which is neutralized by the erector spinae with the sacroiliac joint in the center. This morphological and functional relation is also used when examining the sacroiliac joint with the active straight leg raise test (ASLR).

2.3   Implications for Biomechanics: Premature Degeneration or Functional Adaptation?

Aging brings extensive ridging on the articular surface to the extent that it is present in all individuals over 55 years, as well as the partial ossification of the ISL in 60% of those aged 60 years or older (Rosatelli et al., 2006). It is likely that movement becomes markedly restricted in the sacroiliac joint after 60 years of age (Cohen, 2005; Mitchell and Vivian, 2011). Large variation in joint mobility seems to persist even in the geriatric cohort. Age-related changes start during adolescence and continue throughout life manifesting as the auricular surface becoming uneven, duller, and rougher (Cohen, 2005). After 30 years of age, a narrowing and non-uniformity of the joint can be seen, often accompanied by subchondral sclerosis first on the iliac side then later followed by the sacral side. Older patients also demonstrate a higher incidence of subchondral cysts, erosions, osteophytes, and para-articular ankyloses but these are generally uncommon, even in the elderly (Vogler et al., 1984). Degenerative features of the sacroiliac joint include (O'Shea et al., 2010):

- articular surface ridging
- osteophytes
- dense sclerosis (subchondral sclerosis)
- joint space narrowing

There seems to be a bias toward women although this had no relation with previous pregnancies. There are indicators that overweight patients show more extensive signs of degeneration and that degeneration was unrelated to osteoarthritis in the lumbar vertebrae (O'Shea et al., 2010). Additionally, patients with neighboring conditions such as sagittal imbalance or lumbar spinal stenosis demonstrated more severe degeneration in their joints (Kwon et al., 2020). However, common degenerative changes observed at the sacroiliac joint are not necessarily attributed to pain or functional impairment; they seem to be a chronic adaptation to upright posture and bipedal walking.

2.4 The Subchondral Bone Lamella in Sacroiliac Joint Dysfunction

The primary function of the subchondral plate has been described to distribute loads arising between the auricular joint surface and the underlying cancellous bone (Pan et al., 2009; Leumann et al., 2015). Because bone adapts to mechanical loading, the subchondral plate is also thought to adjust chronically to repeated load transfer through the sacroiliac joint by an increase in bone mineral density (Wolff, 1870, 1892; Kushner, 1940). This demonstrates the effects of long-term mechanical loading, which is also known as 'morphology revealed biomechanics' (Leumann et al., 2015). CT-osteoabsorptiometry has successfully displayed bone density patterns of the sacroiliac joint in painful, surgically treated, and pain-free conditions (Poilliot et al., 2021a; Poilliot et al., 2021b), and demonstrated the relationship between mineralization and bone strength (Poilliot et al., 2020). In the healthy sacroiliac joint, the iliac subchondral bone plate is mechanically denser than the sacral side, and there is a trend toward non-conformity between articulating sacral and iliac surfaces reflecting an unequal dissipation of forces through the ilium and sacrum (Poilliot et al., 2021a). Dysfunctional sacroiliac joints (as described in Chapter 3) yield increasing conformity in particular at the corresponding anterior and inferior joint regions compared to a healthy state. Interestingly, the sacral inferior region shows an increased mineralization in bilateral dysfunction cases compared to the healthy state. This might suggest that this region must compensate for the abnormal loading conditions in response to pain by adapting to the increase in forces caused by the dysfunction of the external structures (ligaments, musculature, cartilage, etc.) that fail to absorb the force as they once did (Poilliot et al., 2021a).

Surgically fused joints also reflect a growing morpho-mechanical conformity, which is likely due to the direct mechanical coupling facilitated by the fusion, resulting in osseous union over the mid to long term (Poilliot et al., 2021a; Poilliot et al., 2021b). Auricular subchondral bone density successfully reflects the altered loading conditions that occur at the sacroiliac joint when subdued to pain or fusion.

2.5 Ligament Alterations in Sacroiliac Joint Dysfunction

The role of the various ligaments in sacroiliac joint pain remains an area of ongoing controversy. Insufficiency, sometimes called ligament 'incompetence', rupture, or surgical transection of the sacrotuberous and sacrospinous ligaments alone causes little change in unilateral sacroiliac and pelvis deformation under experimental conditions. As little as a 30% increase (0.2 mm), has been reported (Hammer et al., 2019a). A larger influence on sacroiliac mobility is observed when the iliolumbar and sacroiliac ligaments become insufficient unilaterally (120% increase), or if all extrinsic and intrinsic ligaments become insufficient on one side (250% increase, 0.5 mm) under experimental conditions. These changes go along with decreased motion at the lumbosacral transition (35% decrease), but increased movement patterns at the pubic symphysis up to 0.8 mm. Of interest, the sacroiliac joint contralateral to the insufficiency shows little change in overall movement (Hammer et al., 2019a). Considering the pelvic ring as a full structure, kinematics changed more extensively if the sacrospinous and sacrotuberous ligaments are affected (80% increase) when compared to injury or insufficiency of the iliolumbar and sacroiliac ligaments (25–40% increase) (Hammer et al., 2019a). It can be concluded that ligament insufficiency alone causes a redistribution in pelvic loading.

Beyond those experimental findings, it has been discussed controversially if morphological alterations occur if sacroiliac dysfunction and pain persist chronically (> months duration). In a patient cohort with sacroiliac pain who underwent surgical stabilization of the joint, it was found that the posterior and interosseous sacroiliac ligaments were partly disrupted, showing signs of loosened and coiled collagens as well as vascularization and hemorrhage within the ligaments (Figure 2.5) (Hammer et al., 2019b). Collagen degeneration has also been found to be an indicator of joint pathology in histology and electron microscopy.

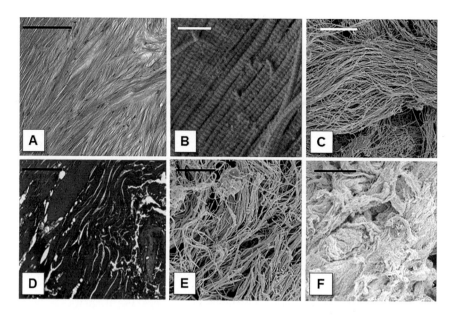

Figure 2.5 State of sacroiliac ligament integrity in healthy and dysfunctional joints stained with hematoxylin and eosin (A, D) and under the scanning electron microscope (B, C, E, F). (A–C) Healthy and intact ligaments showing parallel and aligned collagens. (D–F) Condensed and structurally-altered collagens observed in dysfunctional, painful joints at various scales. Scale bar: A: 500 μm, B: 1 μm, C: 10 μm, D: 0.5 mm, E: 10 μm, F: 100 μm.

References

Bernard TN, Cassidy JD (1991) The sacroiliac joint syndrome: pathophysiology, diagnosis and management. In *The Adult Spine: Principles and Practice* (ed Frymoyer JW), pp. 2107–2130. New York: Raven Press.

Booth J, Morris S (2019) The sacroiliac joint—victim or culprit. *Best Practice & Research in Clinical Rheumatology*, **33**, 88–101.

Buford WL, Moulton DL, Gugala Z, Lindsey RW (2010) The sacroiliac spine—computer simulation of motion and modeling of the ligaments. *Conference Proceedings of the IEEE Engineering in Medicine and Biology Society*, **2010**, 5117–5120.

Cohen SP (2005) Sacroiliac joint pain: a comprehensive review of anatomy, diagnosis and treatment. *Anesthesia and Analgesia*, **101**, 1440–1453.

Dontigny RL (1979) Dysfunction of the sacroiliac joint and its treatment*. *Journal of Orthopaedic & Sports Physical Therapy*, **1**, 23–35.

Dontigny RL (1985) Function and pathomechanics of the sacroiliac joint: a review. *Physical Therapy*, **65**, 35–44.

Eichenseer PH, Sybert DR, Cotton JR (2011) A finite element analysis of sacroiliac joint ligaments in response to different loading conditions. *Spine*, **36**, E1446–E1452.

Enix DE, Mayer JM (2019) Sacroiliac joint hypermobility biomechanics and what it means for health care providers and patients. *Physical Medicine and Rehabilitation*, **11**, S32–S39.

Forst SL, Wheeler MT, Fortin JD, Vilensky JA (2006) The sacroiliac joint: anatomy, physiology and clinical significance. *Pain Physician*, **9**, 61–68.

Hammer N, Höch A, Klima S, Le Joncour JB, Rouquette C, Ramezani M (2019a) Effects of cutting the sacrospinous and sacrotuberous ligaments. *Clinical Anatomy*, **32**, 231–237.

Hammer N, Klima S (2019) In-silico pelvis and sacroiliac joint motion: a review on published research using numerical analyses. *Clinical Biomechanics*, **61**, 95–104.

Hammer N, Ondruschka B, Fuchs V (2019b) Sacroiliac joint ligaments and sacroiliac pain: a case-control study on micro- and ultrastructural findings on morphologic alterations. *Pain Physician*, **22**, E615–E625.

Hammer N, Scholze M, Kibsgård T, et al. (2019c) Physiological in vitro sacroiliac joint motion: a study on three-dimensional posterior pelvic ring kinematics. *Journal of Anatomy*, **234**, 346–358.

Jordan TR (2006) Conceptual and treatment models in osteopathy II: sacroiliac mechanics revisited. *American Academy of Ophthalmology Journal*, **16**, 11–17.

Kampen WU, Tillmann B (1998) Age-related changes in the articular cartilage of human sacroiliac joint. *Anatomy and Embryology (Berl)*, **198**, 505–513.

Kiapour A, Joukar A, Elgafy H, Erbulut DU, Agarwal AK, Goel VK (2020) Biomechanics of the sacroiliac joint: anatomy, function, biomechanics, sexual dimorphism, and causes of pain. *International Journal of Spine Surgery*, **14**, 3–13.

Kushner A (1940) Evaluation of Wolff's law of bone formation. *Journal of Bone and Joint Surgery*, **22**, 589–596.

Kwon BT, Kim HJ, Yang HJ, Park SM, Chang BS, Yeom JS (2020) Comparison of sacroiliac joint degeneration between patients with sagittal imbalance and lumbar spinal stenosis. *European Spine Journal*, **29**, 3038–3043.

Lee D (2007) An integrated therapeutic approach to the treatment of the pelvic girdle. In *Movement, Stability and Lumbopelvic Pain: Integration and Research* (ed Vleeming A), pp. 621–638. Edinburgh: Churchill Livingstone.

Leumann A, Valderrabano V, Hoechel S, Gopfert B, Müller-Gerbl M (2015) Mineral density and penetration strength of the subchondral bone plate of the talar dome: high correlation and specific distribution patterns. *Journal of Foot & Ankle Surgery*, **54**, 17–22.

Malarvizhi D, Harshavardhan S, Sivakumar VPR (2017) Effectiveness of muscle energy technique to quadratus lumborum for treating innominate up-slip sacroiliac joint dysfunction: a single case study. *International Journal of Clinical Skills*, **11**, 65–67.

McGregor M, Cassidy JD (1983) Post-surgical sacroiliac joint syndrome. *Journal of Manipulative and Physiological Therapeutics*, **6**, 1–11.

Miller JAA, Schultz AB, Andersson GBJ (1987) Load-displacement behavior of sacroiliac joints. *Journal of Orthopaedic Research*, **5**, 92–101.

Mitchell B, Vivian D (2011) Sacroiliac joint pain: procedures for diagnosis and treatment. In *Pain Procedures in Clinical Practice*, pp. 391–405. Philadelphia: Elsevier.

O'Shea FD, Boyle E, Salonen DC, Ammendolia C, Peterson C, Hsu W, Inman RD (2010) Inflammatory and degenerative sacroiliac joint disease in a primary back pain cohort. *Arthritis Care and Research (Hoboken)*, **62**, 447–454.

Pan J, Zhou X, Li W, Novotny JE, Doty SB, Wang L (2009) In situ measurement of transport between subchondral bone and articular cartilage. *Journal of Orthopaedic Research*, **27**, 1347–1352.

Poilliot A, Doyle T, Kurosawa D, Toranelli M, Zhang M, Zwirner J, Müller-Gerbl M, Hammer N (2021a) Computed tomography osteoabsorptiometry-based investigation on subchondral bone plate alterations in sacroiliac joint dysfunction. *Scientific Reports*, **11**, 8652.

Poilliot A, Doyle T, Tomlinson J, Zhang M, Zwirner J, Hammer N (2019) Quantification of fat in the posterior sacroiliac joint region: fat volume is sex and age dependant. *Scientific Reports*, **9**, 14935.

Poilliot A, Kurosawa D, Toranelli M, Zhang M, Zwirner J, Müller-Gerbl M, Hammer N (2021b) Subchondral bone changes following sacroiliac joint arthrodesis—a morpho-mechanical assessment of surgical treatment of the painful joint. *Pain Physician*, **24**, E317–E326.

Poilliot A, Li KC, Müller-Gerbl M, Toranelli M, Zhang M, Zwirner J, Hammer N (2020) Subchondral bone strength of the sacroiliac joint: a combined approach using computed tomography osteoabsorptiometry (CT-OAM) imaging and biomechanical validation. *Journal of the Mechanical Behavior of Biomedical Materials*, **111**, 103978.

Puhakka KB, Melsen F, Jurik AG, Boel LW, Vesterby A, Egund N (2004) MR imaging of the normal sacroiliac joint with correlation to histology. *Skeletal Radiology*, **33**, 15–28.

Ramezani M, Klima S, de la Herverie PLC, Campo J, Le Joncour JB, Rouquette C, Scholze M, Hammer N (2019) In silico pelvis and sacroiliac joint motion: refining a model of the human osteoligamentous pelvis for assessing physiological load deformation using an inverted validation approach. *BioMed Research International*, **2019**, 3973170. doi: 10.1155/2019/3973170.

Richardson C, Snijders C, Hides J, Damen L, Pas M, Storm J (2002) The relation between the transversus abdominis muscles, sacroiliac joint mechanics, and low back pain. *Spine*, **27**, 399–405.

Rosatelli A, Agur A, Chhaya S (2006) Anatomy of the interosseous region of the sacroiliac joint. *Journal of Orthopaedic and Sports Physical Therapy*, **36**, 200–208.

Schmidt GL, Bhandutia AK, Altman DT (2018) Management of sacroiliac joint pain. *Journal of the American Academy of Orthopaedic Surgeons*, **26**, 610–616.

Slipman CW, Whyte IWS, Chow DW, Chou L, Lenrow D, Ellen M (2001) Sacroiliac joint syndrome. *Pain Physician*, **4**, 143–152.

Snijders CJ, Vleeming A, Stoeckart R (1993) Transfer of lumbosacral load to iliac bones and legs. Part 1: biomechanics of self-bracing of the sacroiliac joints and its significance for treatment and exercise. *Clinical Biomechanics*, **8**, 285–294.

Solomon LB, Howie DW, Henneberg M (2014) The variability of the volume of os coxae and linear pelvic morphometry: considerations for total hip arthroplasty. *Journal of Arthroplasty*, **29**, 769–776.

Toyohara R, Kurosawa D, Hammer N, et al. (2020) Finite element analysis of load transition on sacroiliac joint during bipedal walking. *Scientific Reports*, **10**, 13683.

Vleeming A, Mooney V, Dorman T, Snijders C, Stoeckart R (1997) *Movement, Stability, and Low Back Pain: The Essential Role of the Pelvis*. New York: Churchill Livingstone.

Vleeming A, Schuenke M, Masi A, Carreiro J, Danneels L, Willard F (2012) The sacroiliac joint: an overview of its anatomy, function and potential clinical implications. *Journal of Anatomy*, **221**, 537–567.

Vogler J, Brown W, Helms C, Genant H (1984) The normal sacroiliac joint: a CT study of asymptomatic patients. *Radiology*, **151**, 433–437.

Walheim GG, Selvik G (1984) Mobility of the pubic symphysis: in vivo measurements with an electromechanic method and a roentgen stereophotogrammetric method. *Clinical Orthopaedics and Related Research*, 129–135.

Wolff J (1870) Über die innere Architektur der Knochen und ihre Bedeutung für die Frage vom Knochenwachstum. *Virchows Archiv*, **50**, 389–453.

Wolff J (1892) *Das Gesetz der Transformation der Knochen*. Berlin: A. Hirschwald.

Zlomislic V, Garfin SR (2019) Anatomy and biomechanics of the sacroiliac joint. *Techniques in Orthopaedics*, **34**, 70–75.

chapter three

Diagnosis of Sacroiliac Joint Dysfunction

Amélie Poilliot, Britt Stuge, Jennifer Saunders,
Niels Hammer and Daisuke Kurosawa

Contents

The sacroiliac joint is increasingly recognized as a cause of pain in patients with low back pain and is typically involved in pelvic girdle pain (Vleeming et al., 2008; Sembrano and Polly, 2009). Whereas low back pain is usually defined as pain between the twelfth rib and the gluteal fold, pelvic girdle pain is defined as pain experienced between the posterior iliac crest and the gluteal fold, particularly in the vicinity of the sacroiliac joint (Vleeming et al., 2008).

Sacroiliac joint dysfunction can be defined as a clinical condition affecting 13–32% of all patients suffering from chronic lower back pain (Nyström et al., 2017). The condition has been recorded in both children and adults with its prevalence increasing from the ages of six to adulthood (Mierau et al., 1984). Sacroiliac joint dysfunction, also termed 'sacroiliac joint syndrome', describes limited function, pain, or other neuropathic conditions in the sacroiliac joint region (Slipman et al., 2001; Clavel, 2011). Generally, the term sacroiliac joint dysfunction describes discomfort in or around the sacroiliac joint presumed to be due to biomechanical alterations such as hypo- or hypermobility, misalignment, or fixation of the joint caused by the failure of the form/force closure system of the pelvis (Freburger and Riddle, 2001). The quality of life for patients with dysfunction is recorded to be worse than that of patients with chronic

DOI: 10.1201/9781003348160-3

pulmonary obstructive disease and similar to that of patients with hip or knee osteoarthritis (Schmidt et al., 2018). The sacroiliac joint, however, is still underappreciated as a source of mechanical lower back pain or pelvic girdle pain (Schwarzer et al., 1995; Cohen et al., 2013; Youssef et al., 2016). Literature is scarce on the subject of the sacroiliac joint dysfunction, because its relevance is often overshadowed by better-known causes of back pain such as nucleus pulposus herniation, pain in the hip joint, and leg radicular pain (Forst et al., 2006; Mitchell and Vivian, 2011).

Sacroiliac joint dysfunction also arises in relation to pregnancy in females, and is defined as pain in the pelvic musculoskeletal system that does not derive from gynecological and urological disorders. A diagnosis of mechanical dysfunction can be reached after the exclusion of lumbar causes. The pain or functional impairments in relation to pelvic girdle pain should be reproducible by specific clinical tests (Vleeming et al., 2008). The proximity of the sacroiliac joint, embedded between the loaded structures of the spine-pelvis-hip complex and pelvic organs underline the importance of performing a proper differential diagnosis (Kissling et al., 1990). Diagnosis of sacroiliac joint pain is often delayed due to a lack of specific imaging findings (Slipman et al., 1996; Maigne et al., 1998; Foley and Buschbacher, 2006; Thawrani et al., 2019); therefore, many patients experience chronic pain without appropriate treatment. However, its clinical features (physical findings) are characteristic. It is possible to suspect pain originating from the sacroiliac joint based on the patients' anamnesis and a well-chosen combination of physical examination procedures.

3.1   Etiology and Pathogenesis of Sacroiliac Joint Dysfunction

by Amélie Poilliot

The causes of sacroiliac joint dysfunction are unclear and probably multifactorial. Possible underlying causes include hormonal and biomechanical aspects, inadequate motor control, and stress on ligament structures (O'Sullivan and Beales, 2007).

It may arise from different mechanisms associated with a current or past pregnancy, etiological conditions, and predisposed conditions but may also arise secondary to trauma (Chou et al., 2004; Cohen, 2005; Forst et al., 2006; Vleeming et al., 2012; Booth and Morris, 2019). These list trauma resulting from a direct fall on the buttocks, a step into an unexpected hole or step from a miscalculated height as being examples of direct influence on the sacroiliac joint. Furthermore, motor accidents such as rear-end crashes with foot on the break at impact or a lateral blow to the pelvic ring from a broadside vehicle accident have proven to cause acute sacroiliac joint pain (Slipman et al., 2001). Repetitive shear or torsion forces on the joint like heavy lifting or sports like figure skating, golf, rowing, or bowling can also be mechanisms for dysfunction (Timm, 1999; Slipman et al., 2001; Kunene et al., 2018). Additionally, continuous imbalanced and unilateral loads may have a direct impact in rendering the strong ligamentous structures and sacroiliac bony fixations incompetent and imbalanced over time, as insufficient or asymmetric compression of the sacroiliac joints were demonstrated to occur in sufferers of sacroiliac dysfunction (Fortin, 1993; Vleeming et al., 2012). For example, athletes in sports using unidirectional repetitive forces on one side like golfers, dancers, and figure skaters have a higher chance of developing sacroiliac dysfunction because of the continuous shear forces transmitted from the axial loading along the bicondylar femoral axis to the hip bones (Fortin, 1993; Marshall, 1995; Peebles and Jonas, 2017; Kunene et al., 2018).

A study by Chou et al. (2004) determined that of their patients with dysfunction, 44% were related to trauma and 21% repetitive injury being the inciting events for the development of sacroiliac joint pain. The remaining 35% had idiopathic or spontaneous onset of dysfunction. Another study by Jesse et al. (2017) showed that morphological variation in the shape of the auricular surfaces may play a part in the spontaneous onset of sacroiliac joint pain in patients with type 3 (crescent shape) morphology. In addition, Ito et al. (2020) reported an increased innominate anterior rotation on the painful side (2.1°, [95% CI: 1.2–3.0]) when compared to the non-painful side in sacroiliac joints of patients with pain. They also determined that sacral auricular surfaces with superior rotation were associated with this downward rotation of the joint. Pain could, therefore, be caused by the tension of the superior part of the posterior sacroiliac joint region.

3.2 Symptoms and Characteristics of Sacroiliac Joint Dysfunction

by Niels Hammer, Daisuke Kurosawa and Amélie Poilliot

Patients with sacroiliac joint dysfunction often present with a short sitting tolerance on a chair without back rest owing to exacerbated pain (McGregor and Cassidy, 1983; Bornemann et al., 2017). Pain can also aggravate when lying down on the sore side, riding in the car, and flexing the body forward while the knees are fully flexed (Bernard and Cassidy, 1991; Slipman et al., 2001). Patients will often find relief when walking or lying supine (Ou-Yang et al., 2017). Because sacroiliac joint innervation is highly complex and variable, pain can be somatically referred from other adjacent nociceptors in the gluteal region, groin, and leg, which underlines the involvement of ligaments as pain generators (McGregor and Cassidy, 1983; Spiker et al., 2012; Hammer et al., 2013). For example, referred pain from the sciatic nerve, piriformis muscle entrapment or L5 nerve root pathology may be directly affected by intrinsic sacroiliac joint pathology, which is why referral patterns may depend on distinct pathology location within the sacroiliac joint itself (Slipman et al., 2001).

Difficulty arises when having to differentiate sacroiliac joint dysfunction from other causes of low back pain, as the pain referral pattern can mimic other clinical situations including intervertebral disk syndromes, soft tissue injuries, and ligament instabilities (Fortin, 1993; Fortin et al., 1994; Vleeming et al., 1997; Weksler et al., 2007). Lumbar disc herniation can cause short sitting tolerance as well, although in patients with sacroiliac joint dysfunction, the pain area in the sitting position is the posterior superior iliac spine and/or the ischial tuberosity in contrast with lumbar disc herniation-related pain areas, central buttock and lower extremities (Murakami, 2018). In addition to lumbo-gluteal pain, groin pain and lower extremity pain/numbness are occasionally observed. These lower extremity symptoms do not usually correspond to the dermatome (Murakami et al., 2017).

An example of a diagnostic algorithm to assess sacroiliac joint dysfunction is presented in Figure 3.1.

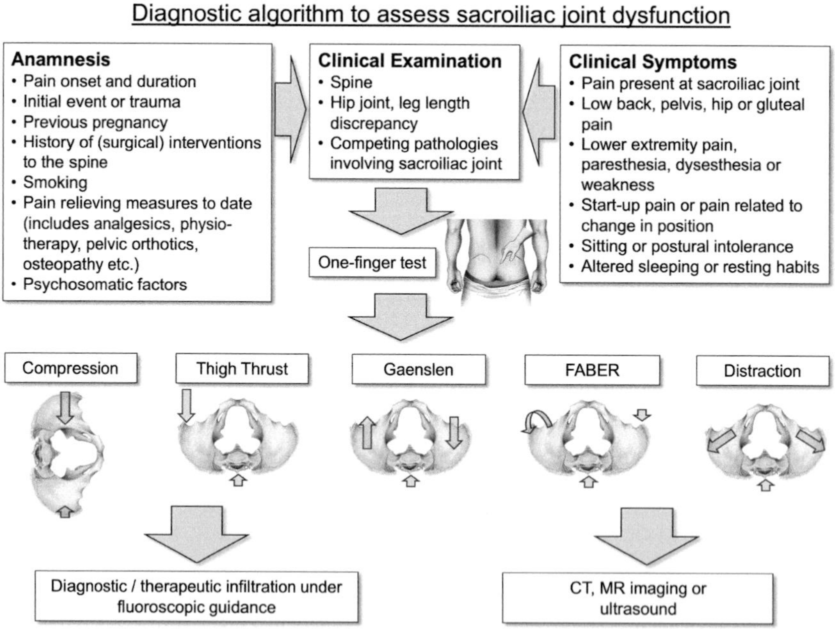

Figure 3.1 Diagnostic algorithm to assess sacroiliac joint dysfunction with illustrated pain provocation tests.

3.3   Palpation and Pain Provocation Testing

by Niels Hammer and Amélie Poilliot

Common diagnostic tests include *palpation tests* such as the positive **one-finger test** (Fortin finger test), where the patient is able to positively identify the painful zone to the sacroiliac area, specifically the posterior superior iliac spine (Figure 3.2) (Fortin, 1993; Murakami et al., 2008). Sensitivity and specificity of this test have been reported as 76% and 47%, respectively (Dreyfuss et al., 1996; Szadek et al., 2009). When other back pain causes have been excluded, this exercise has a high correlation with sacroiliac joint pain diagnosis in conjunction with intra-articular injections (Fortin, 1993).

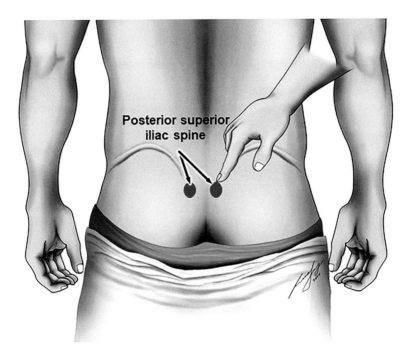

Figure 3.2 One-finger test. Using a finger to indicate painful area resulted in a more accurate, localized identification of the site of low back pain. When patients indicate the posterior superior iliac spine as their main pain area using their index, we should first consider pain originating from the sacroiliac joint.

Pain provocation or *palliation maneuvers* are also used to diagnose sacroiliac joint dysfunction. Common diagnostic tests include (Patrick, 1917; Gaenslen, 1927; Carmichael, 1987; Bernard and Cassidy, 1991; Broadhurst and Bond, 1998; Laslett et al., 2005; Poley and Borchers, 2008; Magee, 2014).

- **Active straight leg raise test** (Figure 3.3)

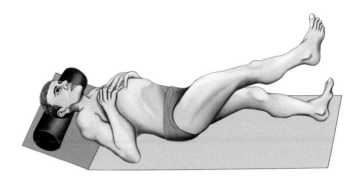

Figure 3.3 Active straight leg raise (ASLR) test. This test assesses the patient's ability to transfer loads through the pelvis (Kibsgård 2017). The patient is positioned supine with both legs slightly abducted. Each leg is raised individually approximately 15–20 cm by flexing the hip joint with the knee joint extended. The test is considered positive if the patient reports a rapid onset of fatigue or pain on the side with the leg lifted.

- **Compression test** (Figure 3.4)

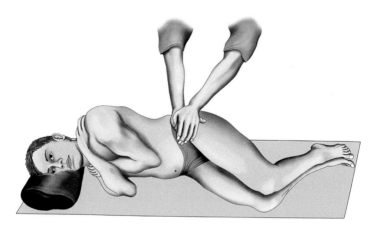

Figure 3.4 Compression test. The patient is positioned laterally on an examination table. The affected side to be assessed is situated on top. The hip joints are flexed 45°, the knee joints 90°. The examiner exerts pressure to the innominate bone just below the iliac crest, directing the pressure posteriorly to the pelvis. The test is considered positive if pain is perceived in the posterior pelvis on the side situated on top.

- **Distraction test** (Figure 3.5)

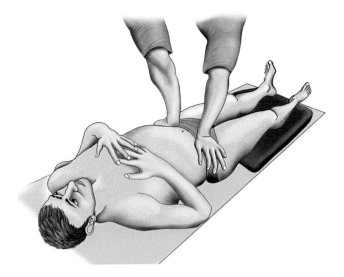

Figure 3.5 Distraction test. The patient is positioned supine on an examination table. The examiner applies pressure to the anterior superior iliac spines bilaterally, resulting in stressed anterior and interosseous sacroiliac joint ligaments. The test is considered positive if pain is felt in the posterior pelvis region.

- **FABER (Patrick) test** (Figure 3.6)

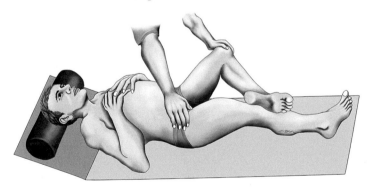

Figure 3.6 FABER test (flexion, abduction and external rotation of the hip joint). The patient is positioned supine on an examination table. On the side to be examined, the hip and knee joints are flexed and the hip joint is abducted and externally rotated. The lateral malleolus is placed on top of the contralateral knee. Pressure is exerted to the knee joint, while the innominate bone on the contralateral side is gently held down with the other hand. The leg position causes traction to the inferior portion of the sacroiliac joint ligaments. This test is considered positive if pain is perceived on the ipsilateral side.

- **Gaenslen test** (Figure 3.7)

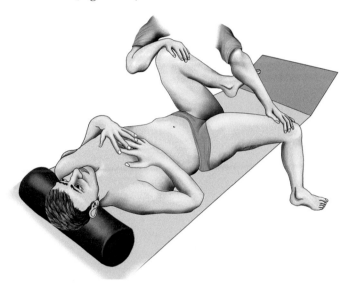

Figure 3.7 Gaenslen test. The patient is positioned supine on an examination table. The leg contralateral to the affected side hangs down from the examination table. On the affected side, the hip and knee joints are flexed passively. The examiner stands on the flexed side and exerts pressure to the hip joint with one hand, while the other hand pushes down the freely suspending the contralateral leg, thereby extending the hip joint. The test is considered positive if pain is perceived on the side with the flexed hip joint.

- **Sacral thrust test** (Figure 3.8)

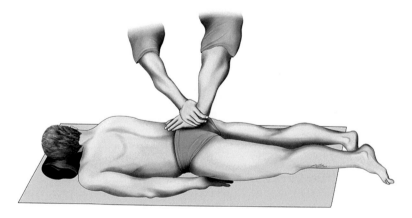

Figure 3.8 Sacral thrust test. The patient is positioned prone on an examination table. Pressure is exerted with region which causes sacroiliac joint pain if the test is positive.

- **Stork (Gillet) test** (Figure 3.9)

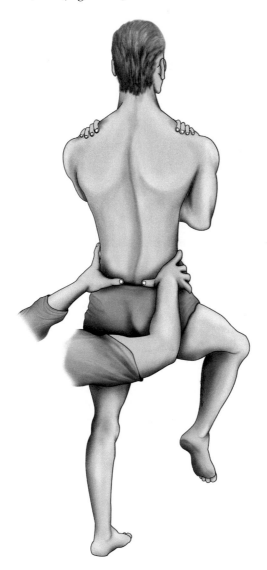

Figure 3.9 Stork test. The patient stands while the examiner palpates the posterior superior iliac spine (PSIS) and the base of the sacrum both on the same side. The patient is then asked to flex his hip joint on the examined side. The PSIS should move inferiorly. The test is then repeated contralaterally, and movement is compared between sides. The test is considered positive if minimal or no PSIS movement is observed (sacroiliac joint hypomobility), or associated with pain located at the posterior pelvis.

- **Thigh thrust test** (Figure 3.10)

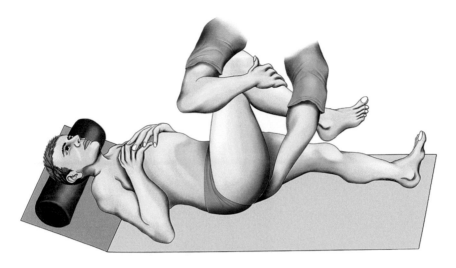

Figure 3.10 Thigh thrust test. The patient is positioned supine on an examination table. On the affected side, the hip and knee joint are flexed 90°. Pain may arise in the hip or posterior pelvis region once pressure is applied to the knee in the direction of the examination table. Further flexion and adduction of the hip joint may aggravate the pain sensation. The test is considered positive if a pain sensation is felt in the posterior pelvis region on the side with the flexed hip joint.

Table 3.1 Sensitivity and Specificity of Palliation Maneuvers from the Literature

Test	Sensitivity	Specificity	References
Active straight leg raise (ASLR) test	88%	54%	**Mens et al., 2012**
Compression test	69%	69%	**Laslett et al., 2005;**
Distraction test	60%	81%	**Szadek et al., 2009**
FABER test	69%	16%	**Dreyfuss et al., 1996; Szadek et al., 2009**
Gaenslen test	71%	26%	**Broadhurst and Bond, 1998; Szadek et al., 2009**
Sacral thrust test	63%	75%	**Laslett et al., 2005; Szadek et al., 2009**
Stork (Gillet) test	43%	68%	**Szadek et al., 2009**
Thigh thrust test	88%	69%	**Laslett et al., 2005; Szadek et al., 2009**

Specificity and sensitivity of these tests are reported in Table 3.1, and the value of the combination of these tests is illustrated in Figure 3.11.

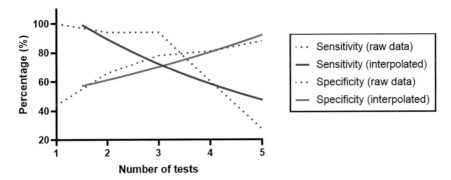

Figure 3.11 Value of using multiple tests based on sensitivity and specificity values reported by Laslett et al. (2005) and Szadek et al. (2009). Three tests show to be the most valuable, as more tests reveal a vast decrease in sensitivity.

Literature suggests that for successfully diagnosing sacroiliac joint dysfunction, three of the following tests should be found positive: thigh thrust test, compression test, active straight leg raise test (ASLR), the Gaenslen and FABER tests *in combination with* temporary pain relief of at least 75% after intra-articular injections of anesthetics (Dreyfuss et al., 1994; Laslett et al., 2005; Szadek et al., 2009; Schmidt et al., 2018; Telli et al., 2018; von Heymann et al., 2018).

3.4 Imaging in the Diagnosis of Sacroiliac Joint Dysfunction

by Jennifer Saunders

Apart from the validity of imaging to assist with inflammatory disorders of the sacroiliac joint, there has not been consistency on the helpfulness of imaging modalities to confirm the diagnosis of mechanical injury to the joint (Tsoi et al., 2019). This chapter will discuss the relevant research and use of imaging to assist with this diagnosis.

Advanced inflammatory disease, sclerosis, and cystic changes may be seen on the sacroiliac joint and or the pubis using plain *X-ray radiography*. There are also subtle differences that will denote inflammatory disease from degenerative disease. This has not been documented extensively in the literature but is frequently seen in clinical practice. These subtle signs have not been validated. Also, noticeable will be some asymmetry of the pelvic bony landmarks (Figure 3.12), and although not diagnostic, give some cues that the bony alignment is not even, hence an assumption can be made that there is asymmetrical muscle tightness around the pelvis.

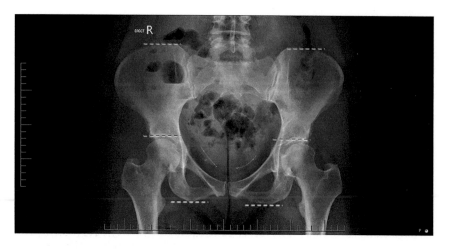

Figure 3.12 Plain X-ray of pelvis showing asymmetry. Lines have been drawn under the ischial tuberosities (green), the femoral acetabula (blue), and above the iliac crests (red).

Melchior et al. (2017) state that the sensitivity for detecting inflammatory arthropathy on X-ray is 82.8% and specificity was 86.9%.

Computed tomography (CT) scanning will confirm bony changes to the joint surfaces in the pubic symphysis and sacroiliac joints. It is also excellent in detecting sclerosis and confines itself to imaging for later stages of inflammatory disorders. However, CT scans do expose the patient to higher radiation doses (10 millisieverts) and are not recommended to use routinely or for follow-up scans.

Backlund et al. (2017) examined the CT scans of 123 patients with clinically diagnosed sacroiliac joint pain and compared their CT scans to those without pain (Cavalieri and Rupp, 2013). They concluded that CT itself yielded no significant difference between the two groups and that CT scans could not be used to confirm diagnosis of sacroiliac joint pain. Ito et al. (2020) looked at 11 CT scans of adult patients and, using a coordinate system of bony landmarks, concluded that this particular system could be used to confirm sacroiliac joint injury. This is not yet a standard approach in CT radiography. Figure 3.13 and Figure 3.14 exemplify non-inflammatory and inflammatory sclerosis of the sacroiliac joint, respectively.

Magnetic resonance imaging (MRI) scans can show inflammatory changes along the edges of the pubic symphysis and the sacroiliac joints. MRI helps detect bone edema at bone areas under increasing metabolic stress. Contemporary research discusses the role of MRI scanning in the diagnosis of inflammatory disorders. To date, little research has been

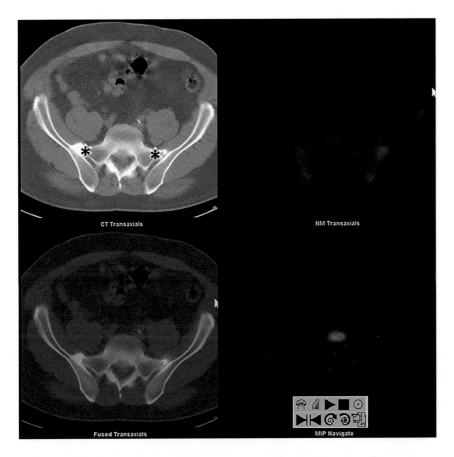

Figure 3.13 SPECT-CT on non-inflammatory sacroiliac joint sclerosis. Asterisks show the sclerosis. CT can be combined with magnetic resonance imaging or single photon emission CT (SPECT).

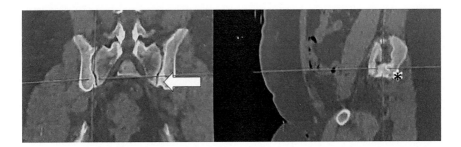

Figure 3.14 Inflammatory sacroiliac joint sclerosis. The arrow points to the sclerosis, and the asterisk depicts erosions particularly seen on the sagittal view in the SPECT-CT scans.

performed regarding the effects seen from mechanical issues of the sacroiliac joint (Hammer et al., 2015; Soisson et al., 2015). Arnbak et al. (2016, 2019) discussed the changes seen in inflammatory conditions of the sacroiliac joint and organized these findings into subgroups. Maksymowych et al. (2017) discussed the MRI changes seen in non-inflammatory (non-axial spondyloarthritis) conditions of the sacroiliac joint.

As the synovial part of the sacroiliac joint is predominantly situated in the anterior and inferior portion, signs of inflammation seen in this area can be assumed to be due to true joint inflammation. This is more common in inflammatory conditions of the sacroiliac joint. Bone edema in the proximal joint in the proximal part of the joint where the syndesmotic ligament of the sacroiliac joint is more indicative of mechanical derangements to the sacroiliac joint (Figure 3.15). Although this assumption needs to be fully validated, it certainly is suggestive given the number of ligaments in this region. The Canada Denmark Working Group on changes in MRI scanning identifies four criteria at review when looking at MRIs of sacroiliac joint joints. These are erosion, backfill (loss of iliac or sacral cortical bone on T1WSE), fat metaplasia, and ankylosis.

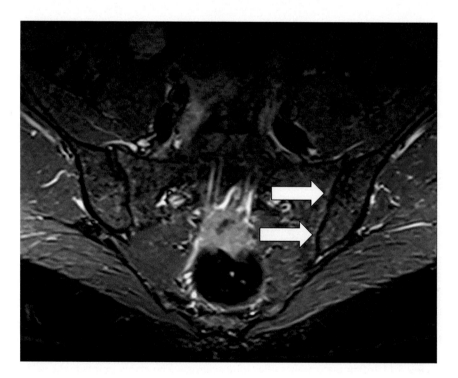

Figure 3.15 Subtle bone edema (white arrows) along the whole of the left ilia surface often seen in mechanical sacroiliac joint issues.

Tsoi et al. (2019) recommend that only radiologists with skill in reading MRI for sacroiliac joint issues should be involved, as there are subtle differences between infective, inflammatory, stress reaction, and insufficiency fracture, osteoarthritis, and osteitis condensans ilii. They recommend the use of a specific scoring system to diagnose inflammatory osteoarthritis such as the Berlin MRI score or the SPARCC score. Furthermore, Arnbak et al. (2019) showed in a series of 1037 MRI scans five subgroups on changes seen in MRI of both the lumbar spine and sacroiliac joint, with those showing changes having a greater morbidity. MRI scanning is also helpful to image other aspects of bone disease that may be present such as metabolic disease (Figure 3.16).

Previously, *SPECT-CT* (single photon emission computed tomography) on bone has been thought to be unhelpful (Slipman et al., 1996).

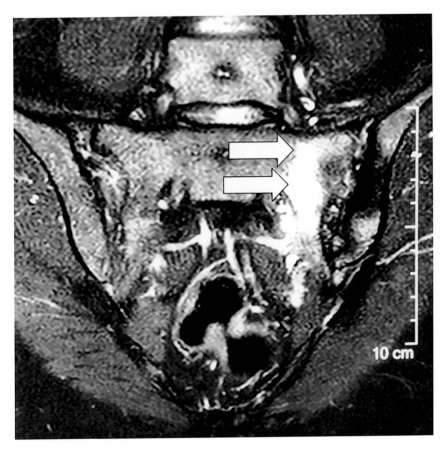

Figure 3.16 Parathyroid disease and bone loss. Arrows point to areas of bone loss.

However, recent studies suggest that when looking at the metabolic changes in ligament-bone attachments, *SPECT-CT* can be reliable in identifying mechanical issues involving the sacroiliac joint (Cusi et al., 2013) (Figure 3.17). The study by Cusi et al. (2013) scanned 100 patients identified by clinical means and compared them to two control groups. These control groups were one group without back pain (being scanned for other reasons) and a further group who had been identified as having nonspecific low back pain. Cusi et al. (2013) were able to obtain excellent validity with sensitivity of 95% and specificity of 99%. This had a positive predictive value of 99% and a negative predictive value of 94%. The power of the test was 1.0 and the kappa values were good at 0.85, meaning the tests were quite reproducible.

SPECT-CT provides pain physicians with an excellent tool to confirm clinical suspicions related to sacroiliac joint dysfunction. Moreover, it helps distinguish inflammatory elements to be observed in the first phase of the triple bone scan and also by the exact place any inflammatory change is noted (superior or inferior portion of the joint). Other structures

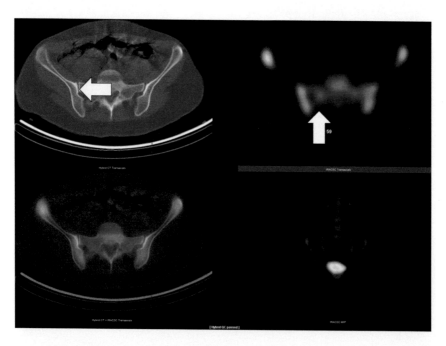

Figure 3.17 SPECT-CT scans show sclerosis on the CT and altered appearance (loss of dumbbell on the bone scan component and uptake in the extra-articular soft tissue).

can also be visualized, including the pubic symphysis and bones, and hip joints. Frequently seen enthesopathies of the hamstrings, adductors, gluteal muscles, and psoas are also noted. Often, these are asymptomatic and are reflective of the increased load on them. Further investigations from our group confirmed the usefulness of this test. Meanwhile, we have adopted SPECT-CT as a gold standard and perform it when there are contraindications to its use. A note of caution is the amount of radioactivity the patient will be exposed to, which is 4–6 millisieverts per scan. A common finding observed in SPECT-CT related to sacroiliac joint dysfunction is that the adductor and hamstring entheses tend to show increased signal uptake. This can occur in mechanical disease due to the ongoing altered muscle function, and the increased effort required by adductors, hamstrings, and hip flexors as they accommodate for the optimal muscle stabilizers.

Positron emission tomography (PET) scanning exposes the patient to much greater radiation and includes a whole-body CT scan as well as bone scan. It is, therefore, thought to be contraindicated and not able to show any more information than would be seen on SPECT-CT scan. Only one reference could be located regarding its use and is suggestive for use in very limited circumstances for inflammatory disease only (Strobel et al., 2010).

3.5   Fluoroscopically Guided Sacroiliac Joint Injections

by Amélie Poilliot

Another gold standard in the diagnosis of sacroiliac joint dysfunction is considered *fluoroscopically guided injections of local anesthetics* into the synovial joint cavity (Figure 3.18) (Broadhurst and Bond, 1998; Liliang et al., 2009; Schneider et al., 2019). If a pain relief of more than 75% is observed after 15 to 45 minutes, a sacroiliac joint dysfunction is likely (Slipman et al., 2001; Thawrani et al., 2019). If repetition of this procedure has similar results under the application of anesthetics, and competing pathologies can be ruled out, this confirms the diagnosis of sacroiliac joint dysfunction. Two techniques of sacroiliac joint injections exist: peri- and intra-articular. Peri-articular sacroiliac joint injections target the sacroiliac joint posterior ligamentous area (Figure 3.18A) and are technically easier to perform (Figure 3.18B) (Murakami et al., 2007). Moreover, given the local concentration nociceptors in the posterior ligamentous region (Sakamoto et al., 2001; Vilensky et al., 2002; Szadek et al., 2008), peri-articular injections may reach the target structures quite effectively.

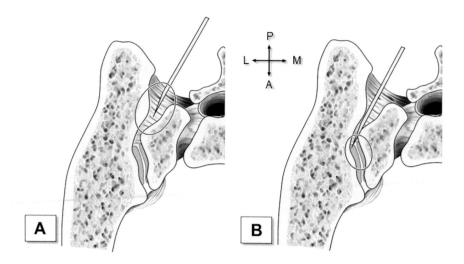

Figure 3.18 Two types of sacroiliac joint injections. (A) Peri-articular injections, (B) intra-articular injections (transverse plane). A: anterior, L: lateral, M: medial, P: posterior.

3.6   Differential Diagnosis of Sacroiliac Joint Pain

by Amélie Poilliot and Niels Hammer

Etiological sources of pain around the sacroiliac region can be divided into intra-articular (e.g., arthritis or infection) and extra-articular conditions (Bernard and Cassidy, 1991; Vleeming et al., 1997; Calvillo et al., 2000; Cohen, 2005; Mitchell and Vivian, 2011). These conditions can be divided into mechanical, inflammatory, infectious, bone diseases, and tumor groups (from Kissling and Michel, 1997):

Mechanical affection of known cause (closely interlinked with sacroiliac joint dysfunction) include:

- sacroiliac joint arthritis
- post-traumatic arthritis
- hyperostosis condensans ilii
- hypermobility, hypomobility
- pregnancy-related dysfunction

Inflammatory (non-infectious) causes:

- sacroiliitis
- seronegative spondyloarthropathy

- ankylosing spondylitis
- psoriatic arthritis
- reactive arthritis (Reiter syndrome)
- inflammatory bowel disease-related arthritis (colitis ulcerosa, Crohn's disease, Whipple disease, celiac disease and others)
- chronic polyarthritis, crystal arthropathy
- other rare diseases: SAPHO syndrome, Behçet disease, familiar Mediterranean fever

Infectious causes (septic arthritis):

- *Staphylococcus aureus*
- tuberculosis
- brucellosis

Bone-related diseases:

- osteoporosis
- osteomalacia
- osteitis deformans (Paget's disease)
- hyperparathyroidism
- renal osteodystrophy

Tumors (benign and malignant)

Sacroiliitis is a common chronic inflammation within the joint and interosseous ligament and is usually the hallmark of early onset of HLA-B27 positive spondyloarthritis (Weber et al., 2010; Mitchell and Vivian, 2011). It can cause referred pain to the lower back, buttocks, and may extend down the leg similar to sacroiliac dysfunction pain (Calvillo et al., 2000) and in severe cases can lead to ankylosing spondylitis, a partial-cartilaginous or complete bony fusion of the joint (O'Shea et al., 2010). Arthrosis of the joint subsequently tends to affect the fibrocartilage iliac side more than the sacral hyaline cartilage side (Mitchell and Vivian, 2011). In addition, numerous predisposing factors can affect an individual in gradually developing sacroiliac joint pain such as leg length discrepancy, scoliosis, gait abnormalities, prolonged exercise, and lumbosacral fusion (Cohen, 2005).

References

Arnbak B, Jensen RK, Manniche C, et al. (2016) Identification of subgroups of inflammatory and degenerative MRI findings in the spine and sacroiliac joints: a latent class analysis of 1037 patients with persistent low back pain. *Arthritis Research & Therapy*, **18**, 237.

Arnbak B, Jensen TS, Schiottz-Christensen B, et al. (2019) What level of inflammation leads to structural damage in the sacroiliac joints? A four-year magnetic resonance imaging follow-up study of low back pain patients. *Arthritis & Rheumatology*, **71**, 2027–2033.

Backlund J, Clewett Dahl E, Skorpil M (2017) Is CT indicated in diagnosing sacroiliac joint degeneration? *Clinical Radiology*, **72**, 693 e9–693 e13.

Bernard TN, Cassidy JD (1991) The sacroiliac joint syndrome: pathophysiology, diagnosis and management. In *The Adult Spine: Principles and Practice* (ed Frymoyer JW), pp. 2107–2130. New York: Raven Press.

Booth J, Morris S (2019) The sacroiliac joint – Victim or culprit. *Best Practice & Research in Clinical Rheumatology*, **33**, 88–101.

Bornemann R, Pflugmacher R, Koch EMW, et al. (2017) [Diagnosis of patients with painful sacroiliac joint syndrome]. *Zeitschrift für Orthopädie und Unfallchirurgie*, **155**, 281–287.

Broadhurst NA, Bond MJ (1998) Pain provocation tests for the assessment of sacroiliac joint dysfunction. *Journal of Spinal Disorders*, **11**, 341–345.

Calvillo O, Skaribas I, Turnipseed J (2000) Anatomy and pathophysiology of the sacroiliac joint. *Current Review of Pain*, **4**, 356–361.

Carmichael JP (1987) Inter-examiner and intra-examiner reliability of palpation for sacroiliac joint dysfunction. *Journal of Manipulative and Physiological Therapeutics*, **10**, 164–171.

Cavalieri J, Rupp M (2013) *Clinical Research Manual*. Indianapolis IN: Sigma Theta Tau International Honor Society of Nursing.

Chou LH, Slipman CW, Bhagia SM, et al. (2004) Inciting events initiating injection-proven sacroiliac joint syndrome. *Pain Medicine*, **5**, 26–32.

Clavel AL (2011) Sacroiliac joint dysfunction: from a simple pain in the butt to integrated care for complex low back pain. *Techniques in Regional Anesthesia and Pain Management*, **15**, 40–50.

Cohen SP (2005) Sacroiliac joint pain: A comprehensive review of anatomy, diagnosis, and treatment. *Anesthesia and Analgesia*, **101**, 1440–1453.

Cohen SP, Chen Y, Neufeld NJ (2013) Sacroiliac joint pain: a comprehensive review of epidemiology, diagnosis, and treatment. *Expert Review of Neurotherapeutics*, **13**, 99–116.

Cusi M, Saunders J, Van Der Wall H, Fogelman I (2013) Metabolic disturbances identified by SPECT-CT in patients with a clinical diagnosis of sacroiliac joint incompetence. *European Spine Journal*, **22**, 1674–1682.

Dreyfuss P, Dryer S, Griffin J, Hoffman J, Walsh N (1994) Positive sacroiliac screening tests in asymptomatic adults. *Spine (Phila Pa 1976)*, **19**, 1138–1143.

Dreyfuss P, Michaelsen M, Pauza K, McLarty J, Bogduk N (1996) The value of medical history and physical examination in diagnosing sacroiliac joint pain. *Spine (Phila Pa 1976)*, **21**, 2594–2602.

Foley BS, Buschbacher RM (2006) Sacroiliac joint pain: anatomy, biomechanics, diagnosis, and treatment. *American Journal of Physical Medicine & Rehabilitation*, **85**, 997–1006.

Forst SL, Wheeler MT, Fortin JD, Vilensky JA (2006) The sacroiliac joint: anatomy, physiology and clinical significance. *Pain Physician*, **9**, 61–68.

Fortin JD (1993) Sacroiliac joint dysfunction: a new perspective. *Journal of Back and Musculoskeletal Rehabilitation*, **3**, 31–43.

Fortin JD, Dwyer AP, West S, Pier J (1994) Sacroiliac joint: pain referral maps upon applying a new injection arthrography technique 1. Asymptomatic volunteers. *Spine (Phila Pa 1976)*, **19**, 1475–1482.

Freburger JK, Riddle DL (2001) Using published evidence to guide the examination of the sacroiliac joint region. *Physical Therapy*, **81,** 1135–1143.

Gaenslen F (1927) Sacro-iliac arthrodesis: indications, author's technic and end-results. *Journal of the American Medical Association*, **89**, 2031–2035.

Hammer N, Möbius R, Schleifenbaum S, et al. (2015) Pelvic belt effects on health outcomes and functional parameters of patients with sacroiliac joint pain. *PLoS ONE*, **10**.

Hammer N, Steinke H, Lingslebe U, et al. (2013) Ligamentous influence in pelvic load distribution. *Spine Journal*, **13**, 1321–1330.

Ito K, Morito T, Gamada K (2020) The association between sacral morphology and sacroiliac joint conformity demonstrated on CT-based bone models. *Clinical Anatomy*, 17–7.

Jesse MK, Kleck C, Williams A, et al. (2017) 3D morphometric analysis of normal sacroiliac joints: a new classification of surface shape variation and the potential implications in pain syndromes. *Pain Physician*, **20**, E701–E709.

Kibsgård TJ, Röhrl SM, Røise O, Sturesson B, Stuge B. *Clin Biomech* (*Bristol, Avon*). 2017 Aug; 47:40–45. doi: 10.1016/j.clinbiomech.2017.05.014. Epub 2017 May 29. PMID: 28582642.

Kissling R, Brunner C, Jacob HA (1990) [Mobility of the sacroiliac joint in vitro]. *Zeitschrift für Orthopädie und Ihre Grenzgebiete*, **128**, 282–288.

Kissling R, Michel BA (1997) *Das Sacroiliacalgelenk. Grundlagen, Diagnostik und Therapie*. Stuttgart: Enke.

Kunene SH, Luthuli H, Nkosi M, Haffejee M, Jooma I, Munro S (2018) Mechanical lower back pain and sacroiliac joint dysfunction in golfers at two golf clubs in Durban, South Africa. *South African Journal of Physiotherapy*, **74**, 402.

Laslett M, Aprill CN, McDonald B, Young SB (2005) Diagnosis of sacroiliac joint pain: validity of individual provocation tests and composites of tests. *Manual Therapy*, **10**, 207–218.

Liliang PC, Lu K, Weng HC, Liang CL, Tsai YD, Chen HJ (2009) The therapeutic efficacy of sacroiliac joint blocks with triamcinolone acetonide in the treatment of sacroiliac joint dysfunction without spondyloarthropathy. *Spine*, **34**, 896–900.

Magee D (2014) Chapter 10: pelvis. In *Orthopedic Physical Assessment*, pp. 649–688. St. Louis, MO: Elsevier Saunders.

Maigne JY, Boulahdour H, Chatellier G (1998) Value of quantitative radionuclide bone scanning in the diagnosis of sacroiliac joint syndrome in 32 patients with low back pain. *European Spine Journal*, **7**, 328–331.

Maksymowych, W.P., Wichuk, S., Dougados, M. *et al.* MRI evidence of structural changes in the sacroiliac joints of patients with non-radiographic axial spondyloarthritis even in the absence of MRI inflammation. *Arthritis Res Ther* **19**, 126 (2017).

Marshall P (1995) Management adaptations for sacroiliac joint dysfunction in classical dancers. *Journal of Back and Musculoskeletal Rehabilitation*, **5,** 235–246.

McGregor M, Cassidy JD (1983) Post-surgical sacroiliac joint syndrome. *Journal of Manipulative and Physiological Therapeutics*, **6**, 1–11.

Melchior J, Azraq Y, Chary-Valckenaere I, et al. (2017) Radiography, abdominal CT and MRI compared with sacroiliac joint CT in diagnosis of structural sacroiliitis. *European Journal of Radiology*, **95**, 169–176.

Mens JM, Huis YH, et al. (2012) Technical and measurement report: the active straight leg raise test in lumbopelvic pain during pregnancy. *Manual Therapy* **17**, 364e368.

Mierau DR, Cassidy JD, Hamin T, Milne RA (1984) Sacroiliac joint dysfunction and low-back-pain in school aged children. *Journal of Manipulative and Physiological Therapeutics,* **7**, 81–84.

Mitchell B, Vivian D (2011) Sacroiliac joint pain: procedures for diagnosis and treatment. In *Pain Procedures in Clinical Practice,* pp. 391–405, Philadelphia, PA: Elsevier.

Murakami E (2018) *Sacroiliac Joint Disorder: Accurately Diagnosing Low Back Pain.* Singapore: Springer.

Murakami E, Aizawa T, Kurosawa D, Noguchi K (2017) Leg symptoms associated with sacroiliac joint disorder and related pain. *Clinical Neurology and Neurosurgery,* **157**, 55–58.

Murakami E, Aizawa T, Noguchi K, Kanno H, Okuno H, Uozumi H (2008) Diagram specific to sacroiliac joint pain site indicated by one-finger test. *Journal of Orthopaedic Science,* **13**, 492–497.

Murakami E, Tanaka Y, Aizawa T, Ishizuka M, Kokubun S (2007) Effect of periarticular and intraarticular lidocaine injections for sacroiliac joint pain: prospective comparative study. *Journal of Orthopaedic Science,* **12**, 274–280.

Nyström B, Gregebo B, Taube A, Almgren SO, Schillberg B, Zhu Y (2017) Clinical outcome following anterior arthrodesis in patients with presumed sacroiliac joint pain. *Scandinavian Journal of Pain,* **17**, 22–29.

O'Shea FD, Boyle E, Salonen DC, et al. (2010) Inflammatory and degenerative sacroiliac joint disease in a primary back pain cohort. *Arthritis Care and Research (Hoboken),* **62**, 447–454.

O'Sullivan PB, Beales DJ (2007) Diagnosis and classification of pelvic girdle pain disorders, Part 2: illustration of the utility of a classification system via case studies. *Manual Therapy,* **12**, e1–12.

Ou-Yang DC, York PJ, Kleck CJ, Patel VV (2017) Diagnosis and management of sacroiliac joint dysfunction. *Journal of Bone and Joint Surgery—American Volume,* **99**, 2027–2036.

Patrick H (1917) Brachial neuritis and sciatica. *Journal of the American Medical Association,* **69**, 2176–2179.

Peebles R, Jonas CE (2017) Sacroiliac joint dysfunction in the athlete: diagnosis and management. *Current Sports Medicine Reports,* **16**, 336–342.

Poley RE, Borchers JR (2008) Sacroiliac joint dysfunction: evaluation and treatment. *Physician and Sports Medicine,* **36**, 42–49.

Sakamoto N, Yamashita T, Takebayashi T, Sekine M, Ishii S (2001) An electrophysiologic study of mechanoreceptors in the sacroiliac joint and adjacent tissues. *Spine,* **26**, E468–E471.

Schmidt GL, Bhandutia AK, Altman DT (2018) Management of sacroiliac joint pain. *Journal of the American Academy of Orthopaedic Surgeons,* **26**, 610–616.

Schneider BJ, Rosati R, Zheng P, McCormick ZL (2019) Challenges in diagnosing sacroiliac joint pain: a narrative review. *Physical Medicine and Rehabilitation,* **11**, S40–S45.

Schwarzer AC, Aprill CN, Bogduk N (1995) The sacroiliac joint in chronic low back pain. *Spine (Phila Pa 1976),* **20**, 31–37.

Sembrano JN, Polly DW (2009) How often is low back pain not coming from the back? *Spine (Phila Pa 1976),* **34**, E27–E32.

Slipman CW, Sterenfeld EB, Chou LH, Herzog R, Vresilovic E (1996) The value of radionuclide imaging in the diagnosis of sacroiliac joint syndrome. *Spine,* **21**, 2251–2254.

Slipman CW, Whyte IWS, Chow DW, Chou L, Lenrow D, Ellen M (2001) Sacroiliac joint syndrome. *Pain Physician*, **4**, 143–152.

Soisson O, Lube J, Germano A, et al. (2015) Pelvic belt effects on pelvic morphometry, muscle activity and body balance in patients with sacroiliac joint dysfunction. *PLoS ONE*, **10**, e0116739.

Spiker WR, Lawrence BD, Raich AL, Skelly AC, Brodke DS (2012) Surgical versus injection treatment for injection-confirmed chronic sacroiliac joint pain. *Evidence-Based Spine-Care Journal*, **3**, 41–53.

Strobel K, Fischer DR, Tamborrini G, et al. (2010) 18F-fluoride PET/CT for detection of sacroiliitis in ankylosing spondylitis. *European Journal of Nuclear Medicine and Molecular Imaging*, **37**, 1760–1765.

Szadek KM, Hoogland PV, Zuurmond WW, de Lange JJ, Perez RS (2008) Nociceptive nerve fibers in the sacroiliac joint in humans. *Regional Anesthesia and Pain Medicine*, **33**, 36–43.

Szadek KM, van der Wurff P, van Tulder MW, Zuurmond WW, Perez RS (2009) Diagnostic validity of criteria for sacroiliac joint pain: a systematic review. *Journal of Pain*, **10**, 354–368.

Telli H, Telli S, Topal M (2018) The validity and reliability of provocation tests in the diagnosis of sacroiliac joint dysfunction. *Pain Physician*, **21**, E367–E376.

Thawrani DP, Agabegi SS, Asghar F (2019) Diagnosing sacroiliac joint pain. *Journal of the American Academy of Orthopaedic Surgeons*, **27**, 85–93.

Timm KE (1999) Sacroiliac joint dysfunction in elite rowers. *Journal of Orthopaedic and Sports Physical Therapy*, **29**, 288–293.

Tsoi C, Griffith JF, Lee RKL, Wong PCH, Tam LS (2019) Imaging of sacroiliitis: current status, limitations and pitfalls. *Quantitative Imaging in Medicine and Surgery*, **9**, 318–335.

Vilensky JA, O'Connor BL, Fortin JD, et al. (2002) Histologic analysis of neural elements in the human sacroiliac joint. *Spine*, **27**, 1202–1207.

Vleeming A, Albert HB, Östgaard HC, Sturesson B, Stuge B (2008) European guidelines for the diagnosis and treatment of pelvic girdle pain. *European Spine Journal*, **17**, 794–819.

Vleeming A, Mooney V, Dorman T, Snijders C, Stoeckart R (1997) *Movement, Stability, and Low Back Pain: The Essential Role of the Pelvis.* New York: Churchill Livingstone.

Vleeming A, Schuenke M, Masi A, Carreiro J, Danneels L, Willard F (2012) The sacroiliac joint: an overview of its anatomy, function and potential clinical implications. *Journal of Anatomy*, **221**, 537–567.

von Heymann W, Moll H, Rauch G (2018) Study on sacroiliac joint diagnostics reliability of functional and pain provocation tests. *Manuelle Medizin*, **56**, 239–248.

Weber U, Lambert RGW, Ostergaard M, Hodler J, Pedersen SJ, Maksymowych WP (2010) The diagnostic utility of magnetic resonance imaging in spondylarthritis: an international multicenter evaluation of one hundred eighty-seven subjects. *Arthritis and Rheumatism*, **62**, 3048–3058.

Weksler N, Velan GJ, Semionov M, et al. (2007) The role of sacroiliac joint dysfunction in the genesis of low back pain: the obvious is not always right. *Archives of Orthopaedic and Trauma Surgery*, **127**, 885–888.

Youssef P, Loukas M, Chapman JR, Oskouian RJ, Tubbs RS (2016) Comprehensive anatomical and immunohistochemical review of the innervation of the human spine and joints with application to an improved understanding of back pain. *Child's Nervous System*, **32**, 243–251.

chapter four

Treatment of Sacroiliac Joint Dysfunction

by Amélie Poilliot, Niels Hammer,
Jennifer Saunders and Britt Stuge

Contents

4.1   Manual Rehabilitation Therapy

by Amélie Poilliot

Manual rehabilitation of the dysfunctional sacroiliac joint primarily should involve manual medicine such as *physiotherapy* and *chiropractic care* to restore normal joint function, dynamic posture control, and extend and strengthen the lower extremities and trunk (Fortin, 1993; Shearar et al., 2005; Polsunas et al., 2016; Prather et al., 2020). Correcting any gait abnormalities and leg length discrepancy should be sought throughout the rehabilitation process (Fortin, 1993). Efforts to restore normal sacroiliac joint biomechanics may include pelvic stabilization exercises to allow dynamic posture control and muscle balance of the trunk and legs. Balance efforts should concentrate around the muscle mass surrounding the joint (i.e., gluteus maximus and biceps femoris muscles) as they exert direct tension and strength on the nutation movement of the joint (Forst et al., 2006).

The goal of first-line treatments rely on eliminating pain generators in and around the joint, and to restore functionality in activities of daily life by correcting any hip and lumbar mechanics (Schmidt et al., 2018). In the acute stages (0–3 days), conservative treatments such as *cold application, anti-inflammatory medication*, and *rest* are recommended (Dontigny, 1985; Poley and Borchers, 2008; Polsunas et al., 2016; Schmidt et al., 2018).

DOI: 10.1201/9781003348160-4

However, therapists should start a corrective exercise program during the recovery stage (three days to eight weeks), which will include *self-correcting exercises* which allow relief to the surrounding sacroiliac ligaments (Dontigny, 1985; Kumar et al., 2015; Schmidt et al., 2018). It is suggested that *manipulation exercises* should begin at the initial onset of pain as to reduce discomfort and progression asymmetries, thus reducing chances of further maladaptive changes (Enix and Mayer, 2019). *Core strength exercises* should be implemented as to teach the patient to use their abdominal muscles for daily tasks as to stabilize and protect the anterior pelvis (Dontigny, 1979). *Impact loading exercises* using a slide board or typical *plyometric exercises* can be used in the final 'maintenance' phase (post eight weeks) to regain confidence and restore strength and balance to the pelvic girdle (Chu, 1992; Fortin, 1993). Athletes or workers with high unilateral pelvic impact requirements will particularly benefit from these as they will enable them to train to maintain a balanced pelvis upon impact and prevent future possible sacroiliac joint dysfunction (Fortin, 1993).

4.1.1   Osteopathic Manipulative Treatment

by Amélie Poilliot

Literature has suggested that *osteopathic manipulation* techniques such as balanced ligamentous tension through manipulation and stretching of the adjacent musculature and ligaments around the sacroiliac joint may be a key treatment for sacroiliac joint pain. The method relies on the principle that ligaments provide proprioceptive feedback when tension is stable within a ligament. Unequal tension distribution can cause imbalances in the joint, resulting in a new 'pathological normal' causing pain. Therefore, altering the strain of these ligaments via manipulation allows the return of the normal physiological range, and proper proprioceptive feedback can be re-established (Tucker et al., 2020). Osteopathic manipulative treatment typically involves a varied range of manual techniques, which may include soft tissue stretching, spinal manipulation, resisted isometric 'muscle energy' stretches, visceral techniques, or exercise prescription. Medical osteopathy is characterized by an all-inclusive approach to the patient, where during a session a complete body assessment and manipulation is often undertaken (Franke et al., 2014). This relies on the principle that the body is a unit with self-regulatory mechanisms where tissue structure and function are reciprocally interrelated (Paulus, 2013). Thus, osteopathic manipulative treatment can be applied to many regions and tissues of the body, sometimes isolated from the symptomatic area based on the clinical judgment of the practitioner (Franke et al., 2014). Osteopathic manipulative treatment is a safe option due to its passive approach and is appropriate to use on pregnant women, hospitalized patients, and patients unable to tolerate active, high-velocity treatments sometimes used in physiotherapy (Tucker et al., 2020).

Osteopathic manipulative treatment still requires further testing in regards to its long-term function (Franke et al., 2014) and its potential physiological 'placebo' effect (Noll et al., 2004). Specific sacroiliac joint targeted exercises are still debatable in their result on pain relief as the motion of the joint is minute, its extent barely predictable, and its measurement is neither reliable nor valid via palpation (McGrath, 2004). Furthermore, inter- and intra-examiner reliability is lacking in this field (McGrath, 2004) as the variability and range of techniques are broad (Johnson and Kurtz, 2003; Fryer et al., 2009; Zegarra-Parodi et al., 2012). Osteopathic manipulative treatment has both positive and negative results in its application. It has sometimes been reported as noneffective when comparing it to controls or 'sham' manipulations where there were no substantial results after the intervention (Rubinstein et al., 2012). However, many studies reported improvement in pain and disability after having undergone regular sessions of osteopathic manipulative treatment (Licciardone et al., 2005; Montrose et al., 2021), and the meta-analysis published by Franke et al. (2014) reflects a favorable result for the use of osteopathic manipulative treatment (up to three months) across the literature until 2014.

4.1.2   Physiotherapy

by Britt Stuge

Treatment, such as *physiotherapy*, should focus on mechanisms causing the development and persistence of low back pain and/or pelvic girdle pain and on what can be done to reduce the pain and disabling discomfort. The heterogeneity of problems among low back pain and pelvic girdle pain patients highlights the need for an individual problem-solving approach. Even though debated, it is unlikely that all patients with low back pain and pelvic girdle pain would profit from the same treatment, and a 'one-size-fits-all' approach to the prescription of therapeutic exercise is not rationally based. It has further been pointed out that patients need to understand why, not just what to do, to facilitate empowerment and commitment to change. Consequently, before recommending any treatment, each individual's underlying mechanisms for pain have to be looked into.

There appears to be subgroups of pelvic girdle pain with different patterns and need for unlike treatments (O'Sullivan and Beales, 2007b). One subgroup presents as being 'inflammatory' in nature, rather than mechanical, as these patients present with constant and disabling pain located to the sacroiliac joint. Their pain might be provoked by weight-bearing, pelvic compression (such as a sacroiliac joint belt) and pain provocation tests. A treatment option for this entity is rest, anti-inflammatory medications and local steroid injections to the sacroiliac joint, rather than exercises. Patients with peripherally mediated mechanically induced pelvic girdle pain have been classified into the subgroups; reduced force closure or excessive force closure (O'Sullivan and Beales, 2007b). Reduced force closure may be secondary to ligament laxity, coupled with motor control deficits of muscles and hormonal influences. This may lead to excessive strain to the sensitized sacroiliac joints and/ or surrounding connective tissue and myofascial structures. Typically, pain is provoked by weight bearing in postures such as sitting, standing and walking, or loaded activities inducing rotational pelvic strain. These patients may be relieved by a pelvic belt, co-contraction of local muscles and training optimal alignment of their spino-pelvic posture. There is evidence to support the efficacy of this type of approach (Stuge et al., 2004; O'Sullivan and Beales, 2007a). According to clinical observation, this group of patients also may gain short-term relief from mobilization of the sacroiliac joints, however this in isolation tends not to benefit in the long term. The subgroup of excessive force closure, however, presents with excessive, abnormal, and sustained loading of sensitized pelvic structures, probably due to too much activation of the motor system. Compression of the pelvis is often provocative, and patients commonly present with habitual erect lordotic lumbopelvic posture associated with high levels of co-contraction of local muscles. Pain may be reduced by relief from muscle guarding and correcting a common belief of an 'unstable' pelvis. This approach appears effective although not examined by clinical studies.

Even though no single exercise therapy has proven to be obviously superior (van Tulder and Koes, 2004), *core stabilization exercises* have grown in popularity (Liddle et al., 2009) and two different core stabilization strategies exist, with controversy about which is the optimal strategy (Brumitt et al., 2013; Bruno, 2014). The motor control exercise approach emphasizes specific exercises for local muscles, whereas the general exercise approach focuses exercises on global muscles (Richardson et al., 2004; McGill, 2007). It has been suggested that therapeutic exercises purporting to restore motor control of specific selected local muscles are unnecessary (Brumitt et al., 2013). However, it has also been emphasized that generic approaches using stabilizing exercises do not address the individual motor control deficits identified in the patients (Dankaerts and O'Sullivan, 2011). Increased co-contraction of trunk stabilizing muscles during tasks that provoke pain and an inability to relax muscles are reported in both low back pain and in pelvic girdle pain (Dankaerts and O'Sullivan, 2011; Stuge et al., 2013). Consequently, interventions should focus less on specific stabilizing muscles and more on daily activities and optimal dynamic control of movements. Inherent underlying maladaptive movements might act as potential ongoing peripheral nociception rather than a strategy to avoid pain (Dankaerts and O'Sullivan, 2011). The examination of daily activities can determine whether the movement and pain behavior are adaptive or maladaptive. With this in mind, *individually designed treatment programs* of supervised home exercise with regular therapist follow-up sessions to encourage adherence and achieve optimal dosage is recommended for patients with low back pain and/or pelvic girdle pain (Stuge et al., 2004; Hayden et al., 2005).

Supervised physical exercise therapy has been recommended as first-line treatment for chronic low back pain for years (Airaksinen et al., 2006). Still, evidence shows that exercise therapy only has moderate effect on low back pain, no clear evidence of effect on pelvic girdle pain, and it seems like one form of exercise is not superior to other forms of exercise (Hayden et al., 2005; Ferreira et al., 2006, Macedo et al. 2010; Saragiotto et al., 2016; Shiri et al., 2018; O'Keeffe et al., 2017). Importantly, exercise should be understood in a context, where the bio-psycho-social perspective guides the prescription of exercise, targeting both social, psychological and physical factors (Hall et al., 2018). The type of exercise probably should be individually tailored to the needs and abilities of the individual. And this is not only about the most appropriate exercise, it is about dosage (frequency, duration, intensity) and delivery (group, individualized, home-based) of the exercises (Shiri et al., 2018; Slade et al., 2016; Hayden et al., 2005). Further, it is about quality (performance, supervision) of the exercise, how the exercise is being performed, and whether the patient needs to be supervised. Two recent studies showed significant and long-term effect of exercise interventions (Stuge et al., 2004; O'Sullivan et al., 1997). In both studies the exercises were individualized, supervised, and delivered as home exercises on a daily basis and incorporated into functional daily life activities that commonly aggravated the patients' symptoms. The study by Stuge et al. (2004) demonstrated statistically and clinically significant positive and long-lasting effects, where disability was reduced by more than 50% for the exercise group compared to negligible changes in the control group. The main focus of the exercises was to improve force closure with coordination of the local and overall muscle system, especially addressing the dynamic control of a neutral position of the lumbo-pelvis, subsequently to develop strength and endurance to manage the physical demands facing each individual. The exercises were performed without provoking pain, which has been shown to be important for adherence (Jack et al., 2010). Patients learned to normalize pain provocative daily life activities, postures, and movements to avoid pain flare-ups. Additionally, essential points addressed were sacroiliac joint restrictions, posture, breathing, and cognitive behavioral perspectives. Cognitive aspects were an important aspect of the intervention, in addition to the exercises. The patients were ordered to perform their 30- to 60-minute exercise program three days a week and they adhered closely to this regime. A qualitative study elucidating this treatment program found that by being active agents in managing their pelvic girdle pain, the patients learned to set themselves proximal goals (Stuge and Bergland, 2011). Perceived hope and self-efficacy appeared to be essential for developing a capacity for self-management and an enhanced ability to benefit from appropriate learning experiences. To improve the quality of treatment, physiotherapists ought to have evidence-based skills, listen attentively, and individualize treatment. The patients found the discussion and individualized guidance as positive factors in helping them to cope with their daily lives. The aim of exercises should be clear to the patient (whether it is about control, strength or endurance), and performance (how) with relaxation to avoid muscle guarding should be emphasized. Adherence may be influenced by the way the exercises are provided (Aboagye, 2017). To promote adherence, the use of patient preferences, with self-defined movement goals, may be a motivational basis for behavior change (Aboagye, 2017; Stilwell and Harman, 2017). The recent low back pain guidelines from the National Institute for Health and Care Excellence (NICE) show a clear emphasis on facilitating self-management strategies (National Guideline Centre (UK), 2016). This guideline suggests that patients' needs, preferences, and capability should be considered. Furthermore, communication skills may facilitate positive beliefs and provide a motivational foundation for empowerment, self-efficacy, and for self-management and empowerment (Stuge and Bergland, 2011; Lonsdale et al., 2017; Nicolson et al., 2017).

It has been shown that *therapy* that is specifically directed at well-defined subgroups leads to improved effectiveness of interventions (Karayannis et al., 2012). Even though recommended, it could be questioned whether unidimensional care such as a 'stay active' approach will target underlying mechanisms of low back pain and pelvic girdle pain. The most effective exercise therapy to improve pain and function in chronic low back pain has shown to be individually designed treatment programs that were supervised and delivered as home exercise with regular therapist follow-up to encourage adherence (Hayden et al., 2005). However, with high adherence to exercises that maintain an inappropriate motor pattern, low back pain, and pelvic girdle pain possibly could proceed into chronicity. Exercises might be labeled motor control exercises, but with an inappropriate performance it may result in stiffness and rigidity, quite commonly seen in patients doing stabilizing exercises. Increased co-contraction of trunk stabilizing muscles during tasks that provoke pain and an inability to relax muscles are reported in both low back pain and in pelvic girdle pain (Dankaerts and O'Sullivan, 2011; Stuge et al., 2013). These exercises may be more about strength than about motor control. Patients may comply with their prescribed exercises; they get strong, but also stiff and rigid and with no improvement in pain and function. *Neuromuscular control* or *core stability* is needed to perform daily life activities, but only low levels of muscle contraction are needed to stabilize the spine (Lederman, 2010). So, when are patients strong enough? Is it a good choice to continue doing the same exercises when the exercises do not reduce low back pain and pelvic girdle pain?

Bending and lifting are daily functional activities which may be challenging for patients with low back pain and pelvic girdle pain. The quadriceps muscle was paid attention to years ago (Trafimow et al., 1993; Hagen and Harmsringdahl, 1994), and recent studies highlight exercises incorporated into functional tasks (O'Sullivan, 2005; Fersum et al., 2010; O'Sullivan et al., 2015). Most functional tasks involve the use of lower extremities. However, it is often seen that patients with pelvic girdle pain adapt to an inappropriate motor pattern where they, for example, reduce using their lower extremities and compensate with the arms when standing up and sitting down on a chair. So, maybe one essential exercise for low back pain and pelvic girdle pain is to primarily strengthen the lower extremities, thighs, and buttocks. The quadriceps muscle exertion is the weak link for the squat technique (Hagen and Harmsringdahl, 1994), and squats can be performed as home-based exercises incorporated into functional tasks. Not all patients with low back pain and pelvic girdle pain will, however, benefit equally from exercises (Hicks et al., 2005; Foster et al., 2018). Hence, patients should be encouraged to engage in regular exercises they personally enjoy with self-identified functional goals and meaningful movements (Stilwell and Harman, 2017).

In conclusion, patients with sacroiliac joint pain should be encouraged to be physically active, and health care providers should help the patient to find the kind of exercise or physical activity that is optimal for each individual, in their own environment. To enhance adherence, exercises need to be meaningful to the patient, relevant for daily activities, individualized according to patient preferences, guided and supervised to secure performance and quality. Speak to the patient's heart and brain and tell them to practice what 'they want to be good at', and no exercise is better than the way it is performed. Health care providers should recognize that there may not be one single source of dysfunction or reason for the problem.

4.1.3   Pelvic Orthotics

by Niels Hammer and Amélie Poilliot

Pelvic belts have proven to be an effective method in improving sacroiliac joint dysfunction during activities of daily living, reducing the load through the sacroiliac joint via the lumbar spine and hip range of motion (Sichting et al., 2014; Hammer et al., 2015; Soisson et al., 2015; Klima et al., 2018; Xu et al., 2020). The exact mode of pain relief is yet poorly elucidated and remains a topic of ongoing research. Potential relief mechanisms may include mechanical tensioning effects, altered neuromuscular feedback loops, and influenced proprioceptive input in the sense of the gate control theory (Melzack and Wall, 1965). There is little evidence of pelvic belts providing efficient compression to the sacroiliac joint as a primary effect of pain relief (Soisson et al., 2015). While the short-term pain relief is minimal, pain-related quality of life is significantly improved in patients with dysfunctional sacroiliac joints (Hammer et al., 2015), and improved steadiness when walking in those wearing the belts (Hammer et al., 2015). Although clinically, orthotic application seems to decrease pelvic laxity, it was found that pelvic belts may anecdotally increase movement at the sacroiliac joint in certain directions all while providing relief to the individual (Sichting et al., 2014; Hammer et al., 2015; Klima et al., 2018). More specifically, numerical assessment of sacroiliac joint kinematics has shown that axial rotation at the joint decreases (Sichting et al., 2014), while, correspondingly, axial rotation *in vitro* at the lumbosacral transition (L5-S1) vastly increased (Klima et al., 2018). The position and tension exerted via the pelvic belt seems to influence the effectiveness of the treatment, however, *in vivo* data on these effects are missing to date (Vleeming and Stoeckart, 1992).

Other orthotic options include *water-resistant tape, cinch-type belts/ dynamic tension bands, three-point pelvic stabilization orthoses* with trans-iliac fixation and *antigravity leverage devices* (rotate the sacrum anteriorly and ilium posteriorly, against gravity effects) (Fortin, 1993; Lee and Yoo, 2012; Neamat Allah et al., 2018; Enix and Mayer, 2019). In comparison to pelvic belts, orthoses such as cinch belts and tape do not restrict sacroiliac joint motion but rather enhance postural awareness and help restore normal physiological sacral mechanics (Fortin, 1993). *Heel lifts* for corrective leveling of the sacral plane due to leg length discrepancies have also been suggested as having positive corrective effects (Dontigny, 1979; Dontigny, 1985; Foley and Buschbacher, 2006; Chuang et al., 2019; Prather et al., 2020). These cost-effective methods can also provide the patient with confidence and proprioceptive awareness after rehabilitation and physiotherapy as their primary function is to reduce sacroiliac joint laxity and enhance pelvic stability (Vleeming et al., 2012; Sichting et al., 2014; Suehiro et al.,

2019). These tools should be used to enhance the rehabilitation process and allow a progressive recovery and return to activity (Fortin, 1993).

4.2   Other Non-Surgical Treatment Options

by Amélie Poilliot

Other treatments suggested in the literature include *acupuncture, electromyography biofeedback training, relaxation training, self-hypnosis,* and *massage therapy* (Slipman et al., 2001). *Extracorporeal shock wave therapy* is effective for pain on the ligamentous attachment site of the bone, such as the long posterior sacroiliac ligament and sacrotuberous ligament, because prolonged sacroiliac joint dysfunction could cause enthesopathy of sacroiliac ligaments due to increased imbalanced local tension (Endo et al., 2020).

If conservative treatments have been exhausted without significant pain improvement or if they have plateaued within six weeks of conservative treatment, other more invasive methods like intra-articular steroid injections, prolotherapy or surgery may be sought (Fortin, 1993; Forst et al., 2006; Schmidt et al., 2018). Results from *intra-articular injections* are usually temporary and can be accompanied by unwanted adverse side effects (Liliang et al., 2009; Hammer et al., 2015; Ou-Yang et al., 2017). Most studies report an average of 50% pain relief for two weeks. Moreover, not all patients receive positive results subsequent to intra-articular injections (Schneider et al., 2018).

4.2.1   Prolotherapy

by Jennifer Saunders

Prolotherapy or *regenerative injection therapy* is an injection technique that uses small amounts of irritant solution into a target such as a painful ligament, tendon or joint to promote growth of normal cells and tissues. The irritant solution is most often hypertonic dextrose (d-glucose), but may also contain combinations of polidocanol, manganese, zinc, human growth hormone, pumice, ozone, glycerin, or phenol (Hauser et al., 2016). In severe cases, autologous cellular solutions may also be needed, such as platelet-rich plasma (PRP), bone marrow, or adipose tissue (Alderman et al., 2011). A major goal of prolotherapy in chronic musculoskeletal conditions is the stimulation of regenerative processes in the joint that will facilitate the restoration of joint stability by augmenting the tensile strength of joint stabilizing structures, such as ligaments, tendons, joint capsules, menisci, and labral tissue.

For those who fail the highly specialized physiotherapeutic techniques, injections into the ligamentous portion of the sacroiliac joint have been shown to be helpful (Cusi et al., 2010; Saunders et al., 2018). A further study has shown that prolotherapy into the synovial portion of the joint gives longer relief than steroid injection (Kim et al., 2010). A recent case series of platelet-rich plasma injections for the treatment of sacroiliac joint dysfunction has also suggested significant efficacy for this treatment (Ko et al., 2017). There are several ligaments of the sacroiliac joint that can be amenable to injection therapies. The interosseus ligament has been shown to be the real linchpin of the pelvis holding the majority of the pelvis together, so it is a targeted zone.

Injections can be landmark guided, fluoroscopy, ultrasound, and CT guided. The choice of technique will be determined by the skill and experience of the operator and the availability of equipment. Generally, landmark-based injections are not recommended as accuracy cannot be guaranteed. Ultrasound represents an economical and good choice as no ionizing radiation is used and has been reported to be accurate (Schneider et al., 2020). A further study showed the efficacy of an oblique approach to the ligamentous portion of the joint (Saunders et al., 2016) (Figure 4.1).

Cusi et al. (2010) were able to show good efficacy of CT-guided hypertonic glucose injections into the interosseous ligament. This technique of a targeted single injection into the ligament was adapted from the prolotherapy protocol taught by prolotherapists (Ravin et al., 2008), whereby low-volume injections of hypertonic glucose are injected into multiple sites around and into the painful joint. This study demonstrated that the majority of the 22% of patients who did not improve adequately with the manual and exercise therapy techniques, were improved with the

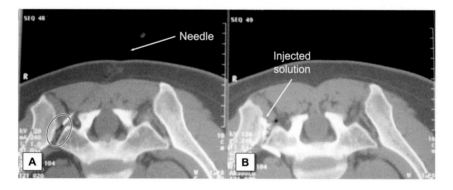

Figure 4.1 CT-guided injection of prolotherapy in the posterior sacroiliac joint space (circled area). (A) Needle placement within the posterior sacroiliac joint space. (B) State after the fluid injection.

hypertonic dextrose injection into the interosseous ligament. This therapy was performed under CT guidance and required between three and six injections to achieve pain relief and functional control.

Platelet-rich plasma (PRP) injection into the same target ligamentous zone under ultrasound imaging has also been shown to be efficacious (Saunders et al., 2018). In this study, the use of platelet-rich plasma to hypertonic glucose injections was compared and were able to show a significant difference in healing time. The platelet-rich plasma group achieved full return to normal function with resolution of all their altered muscle function at 12 months post-presentation, while the prolotherapy group achieved this at two years. Fewer injections were also required for the PRP group with an average of 1.69 injections required, compared to 3–6 with the prolotherapy group. A further case series by Ko et al. (2017) showed similar reductions in pain and improvements in function at 12 months post-injection which were maintained for four years post-injection. These injections were placed into the synovial joint, as opposed to the ligamentous portion of the joint as in Saunders et al. (2018).

Healing and fibrosis then follow the usual tissue healing response (Figure 4.2). The need to warn patients about the initial increase in pain as the inflammatory process that occurs is necessary for compliance. Healing will probably not be noticed by patient or clinician until the four to six weeks post-injection, when fibrosis in the ligament has occurred. Sometimes more than one injection is required. It is suggested that the decision to proceed to a further injection be undertaken after repeat physical examination and an assessment made of the clinical signs that have/ or have not changed. Patients will still need to re-develop optimal muscle function. The fibrosis of the ligament stops excessive movement and seems to allow this to happen.

4.2.2   Cryoanalgesia

by Amélie Poilliot

Other minimally invasive treatments include *cryoneuroablation or cryoanalgesia* where the lateral branches of the sacroiliac joint innervation are frozen using liquid/gas nitrogen resulting in neurological necrosis. It can also be used as inflammatory response within ligamentous tissue as a means of prolotherapy (Kim and Ferrante, 2001; Trescot, 2003; Forst et al., 2006; Yang et al., 2019; Lee et al., 2021). Pain relief is almost immediate and is achieved by interrupting or blocking the nerve endings responsible for the pain (Bellini and Barbieri, 2015). As the nerve cell remains intact, normal function and thus pain can return with time and has a short post-operative recovery (Bellini and Barbieri, 2015). There is currently little

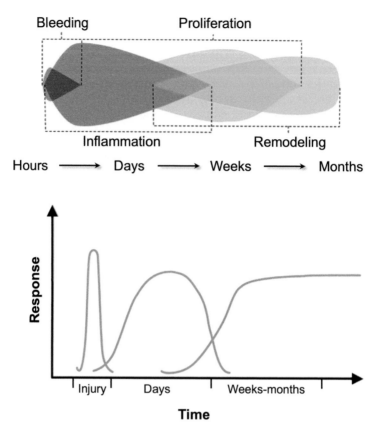

Figure 4.2 Ligament and tissue repair timeline. Prolotherapy has a number of overlapping phases following the original injection and resultant injury with bleeding and subsequent inflammation. Cellular proliferation and repair then occur, with final remodeling of the tissue over weeks and months, restoring partial or complete tissue integrity.

literature published on the efficacy of cryo-neuro-ablation at the sacroiliac joint in relation to long-term effects (Sahoo et al., 2021).

4.2.3   Radiofrequency Ablation

by Amélie Poilliot

Radiofrequency ablation or denervation produces similar outcomes but the posterior sensory rami of L4-S3 are severed or denatured using heat. Under light sedation or local anesthesia, radiofrequency energy is delivered using an alternating electric current via a needle probe into the tissue under fluoroscopic guidance (Ferrante et al., 2001; Vanaclocha et al., 2018; Chappell et al., 2020). Techniques include thermal, cooled, and pulsed radiofrequency. Pulsed uses less energy and lower temperatures than thermal, while cooled uses internally cooled frequency probes to increase lesion size which increases the chance of denervation (Shih et al., 2020). This is a temporary treatment, with limited evidence of this method having positive long-term outcomes over 12 months (McKenzie-Brown et al., 2005; Vallejo et al., 2006; Mitchell and Vivian, 2011; Sun et al., 2018; Chen et al., 2019; Bayerl et al., 2020). Because the sensory distribution of the sacroiliac joint is inconsistent, conflicting results have been reported in the literature. Findings have suggested that radiofrequency ablation techniques have better results than injection-based prolotherapy regarding long-term outcomes, however more research is necessary to understand its use for prolonged treatment for sacroiliac dysfunction (Ferrante et al., 2001; Ou-Yang et al., 2017; Dutta et al., 2018; Chen et al., 2019; Chuang et al., 2019; Yang et al., 2019). In regards to the three techniques, cooled radiofrequency ablation seems to be the most effective after six months follow-up (Shih et al., 2020). It is currently debatable whether this treatment method is worthwhile considering the high costs associated and the lack of prolonged pain relief after a year (Maas et al., 2020).

References

Aboagye E (2017) Valuing individuals' preferences and health choices of physical exercise. *Pain and Therapy*, **6**, 85–91.

Airaksinen O, Brox JI, Cedraschi C, et al. (2006) Chapter 4. European guidelines for the management of chronic nonspecific low back pain. *European Spine Journal*, **15**, Suppl 2, S192–S300.

Alderman D, Alexander RW, Harris GR, Astourian PC (2011) Stem cell prolotherapy in regenerative medicine: background, theory and protocols. *Journal of Prolotherapy*, **3**, 689–708.

Bayerl SH, Finger T, Heiden P, et al. (2020) Radiofrequency denervation for treatment of sacroiliac joint pain-comparison of two different ablation techniques. *Neurosurgical Review*, **43**, 101–107.

Bellini M, Barbieri M (2015) Percutaneous cryoanalgesia in pain management: a case-series. *Anaesthesiology Intensive Therapy*, **47**, 333–335.

Brumitt J, Matheson JW, Meira EP (2013) Core stabilization exercise prescription, part 2: a systematic review of motor control and general (global) exercise rehabilitation approaches for patients with low back pain. *Sports Health*, **5**, 510–513.

Bruno P (2014) The use of "stabilization exercises" to affect neuromuscular control in the lumbopelvic region: a narrative review. *Journal of the Canadian Chiropractic Association*, **58**, 119–130.

Chappell ME, Lakshman R, Trotter P, Abrahams M, Lee M (2020) Radiofrequency denervation for chronic back pain: a systematic review and meta-analysis. *British Medical Journal Open*, **10**, e035540.

Chen CH, Weng PW, Wu LC, Chiang YF, Chiang CJ (2019) Radiofrequency neurotomy in chronic lumbar and sacroiliac joint pain a meta-analysis. *Medicine*, **98**.

Chu D (1992) *Jumping into Plyometrics.* Champaign: Leisure Press. Illinois, USA.

Chuang CW, Hung SK, Pan PT, Kao MC (2019) Diagnosis and interventional pain management options for sacroiliac joint pain. *Tzu Chi Medical Journal,* **31,** 207–210.

Cusi M, Saunders J, Hungerford B, Wisbey-Roth T, Lucas P, Wilson S (2010) The use of prolotherapy in the sacroiliac joint. *British Journal of Sports Medicine,* **44,** 100–104.

Dankaerts W, O'Sullivan P (2011) The validity of O'Sullivan's classification system (CS) for a sub-group of NS-CLBP with motor control impairment (MCI): overview of a series of studies and review of the literature. *Manual Therapy,* **16,** 9–14.

Dontigny RL (1979) Dysfunction of the sacroiliac joint and its treatment*. *Journal of Orthopaedic & Sports Physical Therapy,* **1,** 23–35.

Dontigny RL (1985) Function and pathomechanics of the sacroiliac joint: a review. *Physical Therapy,* **65,** 35–44.

Dutta K, Dey S, Bhattacharyya P, Agarwal S, Dev P (2018) Comparison of efficacy of lateral branch pulsed radiofrequency denervation and intraarticular depot methylprednisolone injection for sacroiliac joint pain. *Pain Physician,* **21,** 489–496.

Endo Y, Kurosawa D, Murakami E, Sasaki K, Takahashi T, Kumai T (2020) Effects of extracorporeal shock wave therapy for entesopathy of the sacroiliac-related ligaments. *Seikeigeka (Orthopaedic Surgery),* **71,** 1263–1266.

Enix DE, Mayer JM (2019) Sacroiliac joint hypermobility biomechanics and what it means for health care providers and patients. *Physical Medicine & Rehabilitation,* **11,** S32–S39.

Ferrante FM, King LF, Roche EA, et al. (2001) Radiofrequency sacroiliac joint denervation for sacroiliac syndrome. *Regional Anesthesia and Pain Medicine,* **26,** 137–142.

Ferreira PH, Ferreira ML, Maher CG, Herbert RD, Refshauge K (2006) Specific stabilisation exercise for spinal and pelvic pain: a systematic review. *Australian Journal of Physiotherapy,* **52,** 79–88.

Fersum KV, Dankaerts W, O'Sullivan PB, et al. (2010) Integration of subclassification strategies in randomised controlled clinical trials evaluating manual therapy treatment and exercise therapy for non-specific chronic low back pain: a systematic review. *British Journal of Sports Medicine,* **44,** 1054–1062.

Foley BS, Buschbacher RM (2006) Sacroiliac joint pain—anatomy, biomechanics, diagnosis, and treatment. *American Journal of Physical Medicine & Rehabilitation,* **85,** 997–1006.

Forst SL, Wheeler MT, Fortin JD, Vilensky JA (2006) The sacroiliac joint: anatomy, physiology and clinical significance. *Pain Physician,* **9,** 61–68.

Fortin JD (1993) Sacroiliac joint dysfunction: a new perspective. *Journal of Back and Musculoskeletal Rehabilitation,* **3,** 31–43.

Foster NE, Anema JR, Cherkin D, et al. (2018) Prevention and treatment of low back pain: evidence, challenges, and promising directions. *Lancet,* **391,** 2368–2383.

Franke H, Franke J, Fryer G (2014) Osteopathic manipulative treatment for nonspecific low back pain: a systematic review and metaanalysis. *BMC Musculoskeletal Disorders,* **15,** 286.

Fryer G, Morse CM, Johnson JC (2009) Spinal and sacroiliac assessment and treatment techniques used by osteopathic physicians in the United States. *Osteopathic Medicine and Primary Care,* **3.**

Hagen KB, Harmsringdahl K (1994) Ratings of perceived thigh and back exertion in forest workers during repetitive lifting using squat and stoop techniques. *Spine (Phila Pa 1976)*, **19**, 2511–2517.

Hall A, Richmond H, Copsey B, et al. (2018) Physiotherapist-delivered cognitive-behavioural interventions are effective for low back pain, but can they be replicated in clinical practice? A systematic review. *Disability and Rehabilitation*, **40**, 1–9.

Hammer N, Möbius R, Schleifenbaum S, et al. (2015) Pelvic belt effects on health outcomes and functional parameters of patients with sacroiliac joint pain. *PloS ONE*, **10**.

Hauser RA, Lackner JB, Steilen-Matias D, Harris DK (2016) A systematic review of dextrose prolotherapy for chronic musculoskeletal pain. *Clinical Medicine Insights: Arthritis and Musculoskeletal Disorders*, **9**, 139–159.

Hayden JA, van Tulder MW, Tomlinson G (2005) Systematic review: strategies for using exercise therapy to improve outcomes in chronic low back pain. *Annals of Internal Medicine*, **142**, 776–785.

Hicks GE, Fritz JM, Delitto A, McGill SM (2005) Preliminary development of a clinical prediction rule for determining which patients with low back pain will respond to a stabilization exercise program. *Archives of Physical Medicine and Rehabilitation*, **86**, 1753–1762.

Jack K, McLean SM, Moffett JK, Gardiner E (2010) Barriers to treatment adherence in physiotherapy outpatient clinics: a systematic review. *Manual Therapy*, **15**, 220–228.

Johnson SM, Kurtz ME (2003) Osteopathic manipulative treatment techniques preferred by contemporary osteopathic physicians. *Journal of the American Osteopathic Association*, **103**, 219–224.

Karayannis NV, Jull GA, Hodges PW (2012) Physiotherapy movement based classification approaches to low back pain: comparison of subgroups through review and developer/expert survey. *BMC Musculoskeletal Disorders*, **13**.

Kim PS, Ferrante FM (2001) Cryoneurolysis in a pain practice. *Prog Anesthesiol*, **1**, 127–137.

Kim WM, Lee HG, Won Jeong C, Kim CM, Yoon MH (2010) A randomized controlled trial of intra-articular prolotherapy versus steroid injection for sacroiliac joint pain. *Journal of Alternative and Complementary Medicine*, **16**, 1285–1290.

Klima S, Grunert R, Ondruschka B, et al. (2018) Pelvic orthosis effects on posterior pelvis kinematics an in-vitro biomechanical study. *Scientific Reports*, **8**, 15980.

Ko G, Mindra S, Lawson G, Whitmore S, Arsenau L (2017) Case series of ultrasound guided platelet-rich plasma injections for sacroiliac joint dysfunction. *Journal of Back & Musculoskeletal Rehabilitation*, **30**.

Kumar NS, Akalwadi A, Babu KV, Wani ZR (2015) Efficacy of adductor pull back exercise on pain and functional disability for sacroiliac joint dysfunction. *International Journal of Physiotherapy*, **2**, 667–675.

Lederman E (2010) The myth of core stability. *Journal of Bodywork and Movement Therapies*, **14**, 84–98.

Lee JH, Chen KT, Chang KS, Chen CM (2021) How I do it? Fully endoscopic rhizotomy assisted with three-dimensional robotic C-arm navigation for sacroiliac joint pain. *Acta Neurochir (Wien)*, **163**, 3297–3301.

Lee JH, Yoo WG (2012) Application of posterior pelvic tilt taping for the treatment of chronic low back pain with sacroiliac joint dysfunction and increased sacral horizontal angle. *Physical Therapy in Sport*, **13**, 279–285.

Licciardone JC, Brimhall AK, King LN (2005) Osteopathic manipulative treatment for low back pain: a systematic review and meta-analysis of randomized controlled trials. *BMC Musculoskeletal Disorders*, **6**, 43.

Liddle SD, Baxter GD, Gracey JH (2009) Physiotherapists' use of advice and, exercise for the management of chronic low back pain: a national survey. *Manual Therapy*, **14**, 189–196.

Liliang PC, Lu K, Weng HC, Liang CL, Tsai YD, Chen HJ (2009) The therapeutic efficacy of sacroiliac joint blocks with triamcinolone acetonide in the treatment of sacroiliac joint dysfunction without spondyloarthropathy. *Spine (Phila Pa 1976)*, **34**, 896–900.

Lonsdale C, Hall AM, Murray A, et al. (2017) Communication skills training for practitioners to increase patient adherence to home-based rehabilitation for chronic low back pain: results of a cluster randomized controlled trial. *Archives of Physical Medicine and Rehabilitation*, **98**, 1732–1743 e7.

Maas ET, Juch JNS, Ostelo R, et al. (2020) Cost-effectiveness of radiofrequency denervation for patients with chronic low back pain: the MINT randomized clinical trials. *Value Health*, **23**, 585–594.

Macedo LG, Smeets RJ, Maher CG, Latimer J, McAuley JH (2010) Graded activity and graded exposure for persistent nonspecific low back pain: a systematic review. *Physical Therapy*, **90**, 860–879.

McGill S (2007) *Low Back Disorders: Evidence-Based Prevention and Rehabilitation.* Champaign, IL: Human Kinetics.

McGrath M (2004) Clinical considerations of sacroiliac joint anatomy: a review of function, motion and pain. *Journal of Osteopathic Medicine*, **7**, 16–24.

McKenzie-Brown AM, Shah RV, Sehgal N, Everett CR (2005) A systematic review of sacroiliac joint interventions. *Pain Physician*, **8**, 115–125.

Melzack R, Wall P (1965) Pain mechanisms: a new theory. *Science*, **150**, 971–979.

Mitchell B, Vivian D (2011) Sacroiliac joint pain: procedures for diagnosis and treatment. In *Pain Procedures in Clinical Practice*, pp. 391–405. Philadelphia: Elsevier.

Montrose S, Vogel M, Barber KR (2021) Use of osteopathic manipulative treatment for low back pain patients with and without pain medication history. *Journal of Osteopathic Medicine*, **121**, 63–69.

National Guideline Centre (UK) (2016) *Low Back Pain and Sciatica in Over 16s: Assessment and Management.* London: National Institute for Health and Care Excellence (NICE).

Neamat Allah NH, Sigward SM, Mohamed GA, Elhafez SM, Emran IM (2018) Effect of repeated application of rigid tape on pain and mobility deficits associated with sacroiliac joint dysfunction. *Journal of Back and Musculoskeletal Rehabilitation*, **34**, 1–10.

Nicolson PJA, Bennell KL, Dobson FL, Van Ginckel A, Holden MA, Hinman RS (2017) Interventions to increase adherence to therapeutic exercise in older adults with low back pain and/or hip/knee osteoarthritis: a systematic review and meta-analysis. *British Journal of Sports Medicine*, **51**, 791–799.

Noll DR, Degenhardt BF, Stuart M, McGovern R, Matteson M (2004) Effectiveness of a sham protocol and adverse effects in a clinical trial of osteopathic manipulative treatment in nursing home patients. *Journal of the American Osteopathic Association*, **104**, 107–113.

O'Keeffe M, Hayes A, McCreesh K, Purtill H, O'Sullivan K (2017) Are group-based and individual physiotherapy exercise programmes equally effective for musculoskeletal conditions? A systematic review and meta-analysis. *British Journal of Sports Medicine*, **51**, 126–132.

O'Sullivan K, Dankaerts W, O'Sullivan L, O'Sullivan PB (2015) Cognitive functional therapy for disabling nonspecific chronic low back pain: multiple case-cohort study. *Physical Therapy*, **95**, 1478–1488.

O'Sullivan PB (2005) Diagnosis and classification of chronic low back pain disorders: maladaptive movement and motor control impairments as underlying mechanism. *Manual Therapy*, **10**, 242–255.

O'Sullivan PB, Beales DJ (2007a) Changes in pelvic floor and diaphragm kinematics and respiratory patterns in subjects with sacroiliac joint pain following a motor learning intervention: a case series. *Manual Therapy*, **12**, 209–218.

O'Sullivan PB, Beales DJ (2007b) Diagnosis and classification of pelvic girdle pain disorders-Part 1: a mechanism based approach within a biopsychosocial framework. *Manual Therapy*, **12**, 86–97.

O'Sullivan PB, Phyty GD, Twomey LT, Allison GT (1997) Evaluation of specific stabilizing exercise in the treatment of chronic low back pain with radiologic diagnosis of spondylolysis or spondylolisthesis. *Spine (Phila Pa 1976)*, **22**, 2959–2967.

Ou-Yang DC, York PJ, Kleck CJ, Patel VV (2017) Diagnosis and management of sacroiliac joint dysfunction. *Journal of Bone and Joint Surgery—American Volume*, **99**, 2027–2036.

Paulus S (2013) The core principles of osteopathic philosophy. *International Journal of Osteopathic Medicine*, **16**, 11–16.

Poley RE, Borchers JR (2008) Sacroiliac joint dysfunction: evaluation and treatment. *Physician and Sports Medicine*, **36**, 42–49.

Polsunas PJ, Sowa G, Fritz JM, et al. (2016) Deconstructing chronic low back pain in the older adult-step by step evidence and expert-based recommendations for evaluation and treatment: Part X: sacroiliac joint syndrome. *Pain Medicine*, **17**, 1638–1647.

Prather H, Bonnette M, Hunt D (2020) Nonoperative treatment options for patients with sacroiliac joint pain. *International Journal of Spine Surgery*, **14**, 35–40.

Ravin TH, Cantieri MS, Pasquarello G (2008) *Principles of Prolotherapy*. Denver: American Academy of Musculoskeletal Medicine.

Richardson C, Hodges P, Hides J (2004) *Therapeutic Exercise for Lumbopelvic Stabilization*. Edinburgh: Churchill Livingstone.

Rubinstein SM, Terwee CB, Assendelft WJ, de Boer MR, van Tulder MW (2012) Spinal manipulative therapy for acute low-back pain. *Cochrane Database of Systematic Reviews*, **2012**, CD008880.

Sahoo RK, Das G, Pathak L, Dutta D, Roy C, Bhatia A (2021) Cryoneurolysis of innervation to sacroiliac joints: technical description and initial results—a case series. *A&A Practice*, **15**, e01427.

Saragiotto BT, Maher CG, Yamato TP, et al. (2016) Motor control exercise for chronic non specific low-back pain. *Cochrane Database of Systematic Reviews*, CD012004.

Saunders J, Cusi M, Hackett L, Van der Wall H (2016) An exploration of ultrasound guided therapeutic injection of the dorsal interosseous ligaments of the sacroiliac joint for mechanical dysfunction of the joint. *JSM Pain and Management*, **1**, 1003.

Saunders J, Cusi M, Hackett L, Van der Wall H (2018) A comparison of ultrasound guided PRP and prolotherapy for mechanical dysfunction of the sacroiliac joint. *Journal of Prolotherapy*, **10**, e992–e999.

Schmidt GL, Bhandutia AK, Altman DT (2018) Management of sacroiliac joint pain. *Journal of the American Academy of Orthopaedic Surgeons*, **26**, 610–616.

Schneider BJ, Huynh L, Levin J, Rinkaekan P, Kordi R, Kennedy DJ (2018) Does immediate pain relief after an injection into the sacroiliac joint with anesthetic and corticosteroid predict subsequent pain relief? *Pain Medicine*, **19**, 244–251.

Schneider BJ, Patel J, Smith C (2020) Ultrasound guidance for intraarticular sacroiliac joint injections. *Pain Medicine*, **20**, 3233–3234.

Shearar KA, Colloca CJ, White HL (2005) A randomized clinical trial of manual versus mechanical force manipulation in the treatment of sacroiliac joint syndrome. *Journal of Manipulative and Physiological Therapeutics*, **28**, 493–501.

Shih CL, Shen PC, Lu CC, et al. (2020) A comparison of efficacy among different radiofrequency ablation techniques for the treatment of lumbar facet joint and sacroiliac joint pain: a systematic review and meta-analysis. *Clinical Neurology and Neurosurgery*, **195**, 105854.

Shiri R, Coggon D, Falah-Hassani K (2018) Exercise for the prevention of low back and pelvic girdle pain in pregnancy: a meta-analysis of randomized controlled trials. *European Journal of Pain*, **22** (1), 19–27.

Sichting F, Rossol J, Soisson O, Klima S, Milani T, Hammer N (2014) Pelvic belt effects on sacroiliac joint ligaments: a computational approach to understand therapeutic effects of pelvic belts. *Pain Physician*, **17**, 43–51.

Slade SC, Dionne CE, Underwood M, Buchbinder R (2016) Consensus on exercise reporting template (CERT): explanation and elaboration statement. *British Journal of Sports Medicine*, **50**, 1428–1437.

Slipman CW, Whyte IWS, Chow DW, Chou L, Lenrow D, Ellen M (2001) Sacroiliac joint syndrome. *Pain Physician*, **4**, 143–152.

Soisson O, Lube J, Germano A, et al. (2015) Pelvic belt effects on pelvic morphometry, muscle activity and body balance in patients with sacroiliac joint dysfunction. *PLoS ONE*, **10**, e0116739.

Stilwell P, Harman K (2017) Contemporary biopsychosocial exercise prescription for chronic low back pain: questioning core stability programs and considering context. *Journal of the Canadian Chiropractic Association*, **61**, 6–17.

Stuge B, Bergland A (2011) Evidence and individualization: important elements in treatment for women with postpartum pelvic girdle pain. *Physiotherapy Theory and Practice*, **27**, 557–565.

Stuge B, Laerum E, Kirkesola G, Vollestad N (2004) The efficacy of a treatment program focusing on specific stabilizing exercises for pelvic girdle pain after pregnancy: a randomized controlled trial. *Spine (Phila Pa 1976)*, **29**, 351–359.

Stuge B, Saetre K, Hoff BI (2013) The automatic pelvic floor muscle response to the active straight leg raise in cases with pelvic girdle pain and matched controls. *Manual Therapy*, **18**, 327–332.

Suehiro T, Yakushijin Y, Nuibe A, Ishii S, Kurozumi C, Ishida H (2019) Effect of pelvic belt on the perception of difficulty and muscle activity during active straight leg raising test in pain-free subjects. *Journal of Exercise Rehabilitation*, **15**, 449–453.

Sun HH, Zhuang SY, Hong X, Xie XH, Zhu L, Wu XT (2018) The efficacy and safety of using cooled radiofrequency in treating chronic sacroiliac joint pain a PRISMA-compliant meta-analysis. *Medicine*, **97**.

Trafimow JH, Schipplein OD, Novak GJ, Andersson GB (1993) The effects of quadriceps fatigue on the technique of lifting. *Spine (Phila Pa 1976)*, **18**, 364–367.

Trescot AM (2003) Cryoanalgesia in interventional pain management. *Pain Physician*, **6**, 345–360.

Tucker DJ, Dasar Y, Vilella RC (2020) Osteopathic manipulative treatment: BLT/LAS procedure—pelvic dysfunctions. In *StatPearls*. Treasure Island, FL: StatPearls Publishing LLC.

Vallejo R, Benyamin RM, Kramer J, Stanton G, Joseph NJ (2006) Pulsed radiofrequency denervation for the treatment of sacroiliac joint syndrome. *Pain Medicine*, **7**, 429–434.

Vanaclocha V, Herrera JM, Saiz-Sapena N, Rivera-Paz M, Verdu-Lopez F (2018) Minimally invasive sacroiliac joint fusion, radiofrequency denervation, and conservative management for sacroiliac joint pain: 6-year comparative case series. *Neurosurgery*, **82**, 48–55.

van Tulder M, Koes B (2004) Low back pain (acute). *Clinical Evidence*, **12**, 1643–1658.

Vleeming A, Schuenke M, Masi A, Carreiro J, Danneels L, Willard F (2012) The sacroiliac joint: an overview of its anatomy, function and potential clinical implications. *Journal of Anatomy*, **221**, 537–567.

Vleeming A, Stoeckart R (1992) An integrated therapy for peripartum pelvic instability: a study of the biomechanical effects of pelvic belts. *American Journal of Obstetrics and Gynecology*, **166**, 1243–1247.

Xu Z, Li Y, Zhang S, et al. (2020) A finite element analysis of sacroiliac joint displacements and ligament strains in response to three manipulations. *BMC Musculoskeletal Disorders*, **21**, 709.

Yang AJ, McCormick ZL, Zheng PZ, Schneider BJ (2019) Radiofrequency ablation for posterior sacroiliac joint complex pain: a narrative review. *Physical Medicine and Rehabilitation*, **11**, S105–S113.

Zegarra-Parodi R, Dey M, Krief G (2012) Traitement ostéopathique de patients souffrant de lombalgies chroniques communes. *Douleurs: Evaluation—Diagnostic—Traitement*, **13**, 17–24.

chapter five

Sacroiliac Joint Surgery

by Daisuke Kurosawa and Julius Dengler

Contents

If all prior non-surgical treatments have failed, *sacroiliac joint arthrodesis* may be sought, although it is more controversial for the treatment of chronic, non-traumatic, and intractable sacroiliac joint pain (Forst et al., 2006; Schenker et al., 2019). Surgery is invasive, expensive, and can have high complication rates (Schütz and Grob, 2006; Schoell et al., 2016; Spain and Holt, 2017). In a well-defined cohort of patients with therapy refractory sacroiliac joint pain, arthrodesis may provide longer-lasting pain-relieving effects for joint dysfunction (Polly et al., 2015; Polly et al., 2016; Fuchs and Ruhl, 2018; Dengler et al., 2019). Fusion of the sacroiliac joint was found to significantly reduce movement at the joint by <50% in all three planes (Lindsey et al., 2015; Galbusera et al., 2020). Minimally invasive sacroiliac joint fusion appears to have advantageous results when compared to open surgery (Keating et al., 1995; Booth and Morris, 2019; Yson et al., 2019; Martin et al., 2020). Regarding the outcomes, studies have shown that surgery results in higher complication rates and an increased risk of infection, but does have better results than non-surgical management treatments for patients which are unresponsive to conservative treatments (Ashman et al., 2010; Polly et al., 2015; Vanaclocha et al., 2018; Booth and Morris, 2019).

Various surgical procedures of sacroiliac joint arthrodesis are performed worldwide with minimally invasive techniques. Of these, three

DOI: 10.1201/9781003348160-5

main approaches can presently be found: anterior, posterior, and lateral. In conjunction, the implants used can vary. These include pedicle screws, plates, cylinder cages, triangular implants, or trans-articular screws and distraction arthrodesis.

5.1   Anterior Approach

by Daisuke Kurosawa

5.1.1   Equipment and Pre-Operative Planning

Subsequent to the exposure of the sacroiliac joint via the anterior approach, following curettage of the joint space, cancellous bone harvested from the iliac bone is grafted in the joint defect before the joint is surgically fixed, for example with a *plate* and *screws* (Figure 5.1). Screws reaching from the sacrum to the ilium enhance the primary stability of the sacroiliac joint (Figure 5.2). A plate placed on the upper anterior part of the sacroiliac joint is thought to aid in effectively suppressing the rotation of the joint.

5.1.2   Surgical Procedure

Anterior fixation of the sacroiliac joint is usually performed subperiosteally, similar to the approach used for open reduction and internal fixation in patients with pelvic fracture; the iliac muscle is separated from the ilium in order to reach the anterior surface of the sacroiliac joint. Dr. Murakami introduced the para-rectal approach for this purpose instead of the conventional one. For the *para-rectal approach*, the patient is placed in a supine position. After positioning the hip and knee joints flexed on the affected side, a longitudinal incision is made along the lateral border of the rectus abdominis muscle over the line of the sacroiliac joint (Figure 5.3A). The external and internal oblique and transverse abdominal muscles are then incised. Then, the anterior surface of the sacroiliac joint is exposed at the interval between the psoas major and iliacus muscles (Figure 5.3B) (Murakami et al., 2018). The femoral nerve should be retracted laterally together with the iliacus muscle, as the motor branches of the femoral nerve course laterally to it. The corridor of the anterior approach to the sacroiliac joint is in proximity to the anterior branches of the L4 and L5 roots (Bai et al., 2018), although usually the nerve roots are not exposed on the sacral side. It is usually unnecessary to detach the iliacus from the iliac bone using this approach.

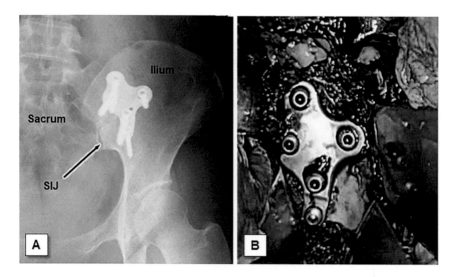

Figure 5.1 (A) Post-operative radiograph with the implant in place. (B) Fixation with a plate and screws after bone grafting in situ. SIJ: sacroiliac joint.

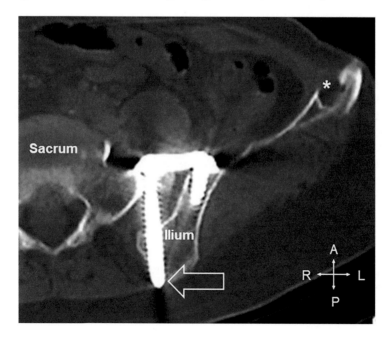

Figure 5.2 Bone harvesting and the direction of the screws on the sacrum. Cancellous bone used for joint grafting is harvested from the iliac bone (*). The tip of inserted screws on the sacral side reaches the ilium (arrow). A: anterior, L: left, P: posterior, R: right.

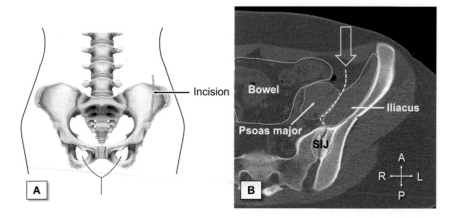

Figure 5.3 Anterior approach. (A) Para-rectal approach. (B) Extra-peritoneal exposure of the anterior surface of the sacroiliac joint between the psoas major muscle and iliac muscle represented on a CT scan. A: anterior, L: left, P: posterior, R: right, SIJ: sacroiliac joint.

So far, the anterior approach to fuse the sacroiliac joint has been used in a Japanese hospital setting in 45 patients with sacroiliac joint pain (Murakami et al., 2018). This approach is effective to fix the synovial part of the sacroiliac joint anteriorly, which is the most burdensome and degenerative part of the joint (Wise and Dall, 2008; Dengler et al., 2019). Additionally, it has rendered being effective to shave the joint cartilage fully using a curette before grafting cancellous bone into the anterior joint space under direct vision. Surgical outcomes of sacroiliac joint arthrodesis via the anterior approach are good (Murakami et al., 2018).

5.1.3   Associated Risks

This procedure is challenging owing the invasive intra-pelvic approach. Further, this access is complicated in obese patients, as the intervention site lies deep to the abdominal wall surface. Third, pubic symphysis pain could occur after bilateral anterior fixation, and may then require additional fixation (Figure 5.4). Post-operative transient femoral neuralgia due to the intraoperative traction may occur. Complications of this approach may include surgical revision and decompression due to prolonged femoral neuralgia with adhesions.

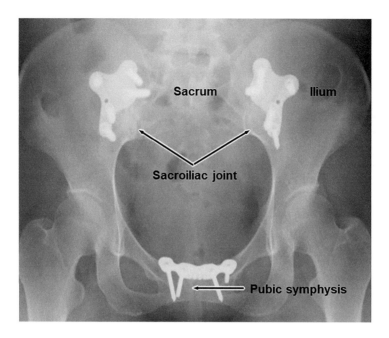

Figure 5.4 Pubic symphysis fixation in addition to a bilateral anterior fixation procedure.

5.2 Posterior Approach: Arthrodesis with PSIS Penetrating Technique for the Preservation of the Posterior Ligaments

by Daisuke Kurosawa

5.2.1 Equipment and Pre-Operative Planning

In order to avoid the risks characteristic for the anterior approach, the posterior fixation technique using an S1 pedicle screw, two S2 alar-iliac screws and cylinder cages was developed. These screws are used widely in spine surgery. Cylinder cages are inserted for anterior superior sacroiliac joint fusion via posterior. In the pre-operative planning of the insertion angle of the cylinder cage, it is difficult to determine the angle because the sacroiliac joint surface appears undulating in the normal axial CT images. The axial images that are created according to the assumed S1 pedicle screw insertion angle, the sacroiliac joint surface line straightens and the pre-operative planning of the cylinder cage insertion angle becomes easier.

5.2.2   Surgical Procedure

In *posterior fixation*, with the patient positioned prone, a paramedian incision is made from the L5/S1 facet joint, slightly distal to the S1 dorsal foramen (Figure 5.5).

For sacroiliac joint fixation via the posterior approach, an S1 *pedicle screw* is inserted into the sacrum, and the tip of the screw is pointed at the sacral promontory, the region with the highest bone strength. Two S2 alar-iliac screws are inserted into the iliac bone to effectively suppress the rotation in the sacroiliac joint. These screws are connected with *rods*. Alternatively, to fix the upper sacroiliac joint region, two cancellous bone-filled *cylinder cages* are inserted in the anterior superior part of the sacroiliac surface, preserving the posterior sacroiliac ligaments largely by making two bone holes in the posterior superior iliac spine, which was modified technique of Wise and Dall (Figure 5.6A, B) (Wise and Dall, 2008). The cylinder cages are then placed from the iliac side toward the sacrum (Figure 5.6C, D). Note that on the radiograph, the placement depth of the cylinder cage is not anterior to the iliac cortical density superimposed line (Figure 5.7).

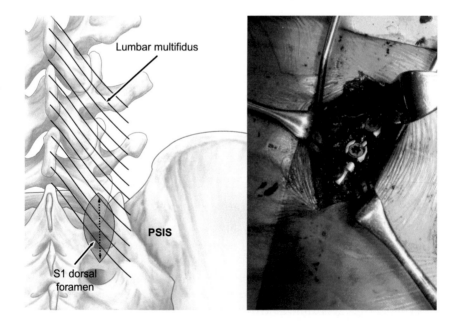

Figure 5.5 Posterior approach. (Left) A paramedian incision (dotted arrow) is made from where an L5/S1 facet joint is located, close to the S1 dorsal foramen. The window for the intervention is highlighted in red. (Right) The posterior approach *in situ* with visible screws in place. PSIS: posterior superior iliac spine.

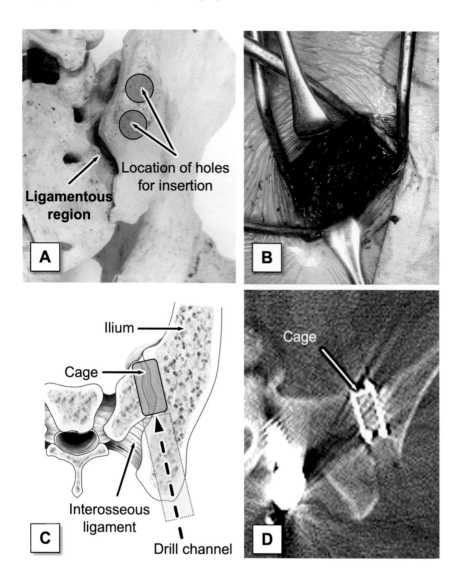

Figure 5.6 Fixation of upper part of the sacroiliac articular region via the posterior approach. (A) Bone holes are made on the posterior superior iliac spine to preserve the posterior sacroiliac ligaments. (B) Screw placement *in situ*. (C) Insertion of a cylinder cage. (D) CT scan showing a cylinder cage inserted from the ilium to the sacrum.

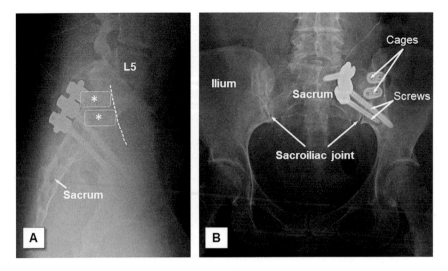

Figure 5.7 (A) Cylinder cages (*) should not be inserted anterior to the iliac cortical density superimposed line (dotted line) as seen on the lateral fluoroscopic view. (B) Post-surgical radiograph (anterior view).

5.2.3   Associated Risks

Because the sacral part of the multifidus muscle runs obliquely, it is unavoidably incised in this area. The sacral multifidus muscles are mainly injured by this approach. Several patients reported pain in the region of the multifidus muscles post-operatively when contracting which was partly relieved by taping to support the contraction of the multifidus muscles.

5.3   *Posterior Approach: Distraction Interference Technique*

by Julius Dengler

The *distraction interference arthrodesis with neurovascular anticipation* (e.g., DIANA® implant, SIGNUS Medizintechnik GmbH, Germany) is an alternative technique of sacroiliac joint fusion conducted via a posterior approach (Fuchs and Ruhl, 2018). It not only introduces bone graft into the joint to facilitate a true bony fusion but also creates distraction within the posterior recess and thereby exerts compression on the anterior area of the sacroiliac joint.

5.3.1 Equipment and Pre-Operative Planning

Pre-operative CT or MRI of the sacroiliac joint help detect anatomical variations or areas of pre-existing ankylosis. C-arm fluoroscopy is required, as are guide pins, a helical distraction instrument, and the implants themselves: fenestrated hollow tapered titanium screws in different sizes that can be filled with bone graft or bone substitute. Patient positioning is prone. The following fluoroscopic views are necessary: lateral, AP, and oblique. The skin incision is marked on the midline at the cranial border of the sacrum on lateral view.

5.3.2 Surgical Procedure

After skin incision, the thoracolumbar fascia is opened about two centimeters medial to the posterior superior iliac spine. The dorsal ligaments of the posterior recess of the sacroiliac joint are partially resected. Using a drill, the cortical bone of the iliac and sacral surfaces is removed. A guide pin is introduced into the sacroiliac joint guided by all three fluoroscopy views mentioned previously to ensure its intra-articular position. The helical distraction instrument is advanced via the guide pin to establish distraction and to assess implant size. Finally, the hollow distraction screw is implanted into the posterior recess and filled with bone graft or substitute as seen in Figure 5.8.

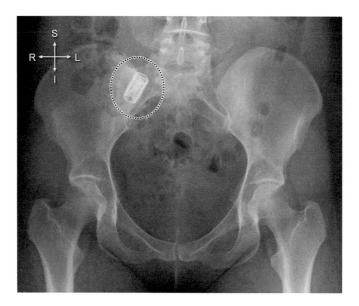

Figure 5.8 X-ray (anteroposterior view) of a right-sided distraction interference arthrodesis of the sacroiliac joint. Implant is circled. I: inferior, L: left, R: right, S: superior.

5.3.3   Associated Risks

During preparation there is a risk of injury to the medial cluneal nerves and resulting paranesthesia in the buttock. Other risks include hematoma and infection.

5.4   Lateral Approach

by Julius Dengler

The *lateral fixation* of the sacroiliac joint using screws or triangular titanium implants is, strictly speaking, not a true arthrodesis procedure, since it does not include the placement of bone graft material into the sacroiliac joint (Dengler et al., 2019). However, a graft transplant into the joint may be added to establish a true arthrodesis. Also, it is worth mentioning that in the process of placing triangular titanium implants across the sacroiliac joint, iliac bone material may adhere to the titanium implants and travel into the joint, so that arguably a certain degree of 'autografting' of bone into the joint takes place.

5.4.1   Equipment and Pre-Operative Planning

Lateral sacroiliac screws are usually placed during a minimally invasive access. They are most frequently applied in the treatment of sacral or pelvic trauma, but they can also be inserted into the sacroiliac joint to decrease the range of motion in the management of sacroiliac joint pain. Over recent years, *triangular titanium implants* (e.g, iFuse implant system, SIBone®, Inc., San Jose, CA, USA) have become the most prevalent minimally invasive device for sacroiliac joint fixation/fusion in the management of degenerative sacroiliac pain mainly because clinical evidence published on these implants substantially outnumbers that on similar implants. Additionally, the only randomized controlled trials available for lateral sacroiliac joint devices to date both exclusively examined triangular titanium implants and showed long-term superiority to conservative management (Polly et al., 2016; Dengler et al., 2019). The triangular shape is believed to decrease rotational forces and the risk of implant loosening.

Pre-surgical evaluation using CT or MRI images may be helpful in appreciating anatomical variations of the sacroiliac joint or pre-existing sacroiliac ankylosis. Equipment required for surgery includes intraoperative fluoroscopy using at least a C-arm, guide wires, a tube-shaped tissue protector, a cannulated drill, and cannulated screws with matching washers, or triangular titanium implants. Intraoperative navigation is helpful but not necessary.

5.4.2 Surgical Procedure

Patient positioning may be prone or supine. Three separate fluoroscopic views are required: lateral, pelvic outlet, and pelvic inlet (Figure 5.9). Patient positioning needs to be optimized using the lateral view with the ultimate goal to align both ala lines until they become one bold line (Figure 5.10). That line then represents the cranial border of the sacroiliac joint. Once an optimal lateral view is established, the optimal sacroiliac screw placement can be located. Over that point, the skin incision is marked (Figure 5.11).

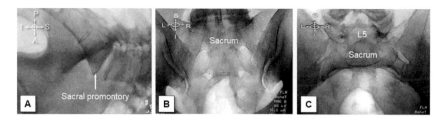

Figure 5.9 Fluoroscopy of the sacroiliac joint. (A) Lateral view, (B) pelvic outlet, and (C) pelvic inlet. A: anterior, I: inferior, L: left, P: posterior, R: right, S: superior.

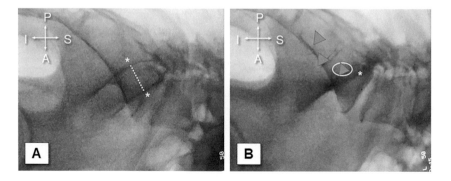

Figure 5.10 Lateral fluoroscopy of the sacroiliac joint. (A) Doubling of the sacral ala line (*) indicates suboptimal patient positioning. (B) By repositioning the patient on the operating table, both ala lines (*) become one and the optimal entry point for a screw (circle) or triangular titanium implants (triangles). A: anterior, I: inferior, P: posterior, S: superior.

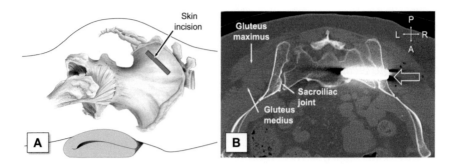

Figure 5.11 (A) Lateral approach incision. (B) Intervention site through the gluteus maximus and medius muscles to reach the sacroiliac joint implant site (arrow) represented on a CT scan provided by Dr. Daisuke Kurosawa.

Screw Placement

Using the lateral view, a guide wire is advanced through the gluteus maximus and medius muscles into the ilium for about one centimeter at the point of screw entry. The inlet and outlet views are then used to make sure the wire trajectory will not breach the anterior wall of the sacrum (inlet) or any of the sacral neuroforamina (outlet). Using the outlet and inlet views, the guide wire is advanced to the desired depth across the joint into the sacrum. In case of a second screw, a second guide wire needs to be placed at least one centimeter caudal to the first using the same technique. Usually, the first guide wire can be advanced through the entire sacrum into the contralateral ilium for bilateral fixation, using inlet and outlet views in the process. For actual screw placement, a tissue protector is placed over the guide wire. Using a drill, a canal is created across the joint into the sacrum. Then, screws are outfitted with a washer and placed along the guide wire into the sacrum to the desired depth. In case of poor bone quality, cement augmentation can be considered.

Placement of Triangular Titanium Implants

In the case of triangular titanium implant placement (Figure 5.12) the skin incision is marked roughly in the middle of all three implants. After the skin incision, the guide wires for the first two implants are advanced at their points of entry into the ilium at an initial depth of about one centimeter. Inlet and outlet views are used to verify that the expected trajectory will not breach the anterior wall of the sacrum (inlet) or any of the sacral neuroforamina (outlet). Using the same views, the guide wires are advanced to the desired depth across the joint into the sacrum. The guide wire for the first implant is usually advanced deeper than the wires for the other implants. Next, the tissue protector is inserted over the wire and a cannulated drill is used to burr across the joint into the sacrum. The canals are broadened into a triangular shape using the triangular chisel slightly across the joint into the sacrum. The first two implants are placed

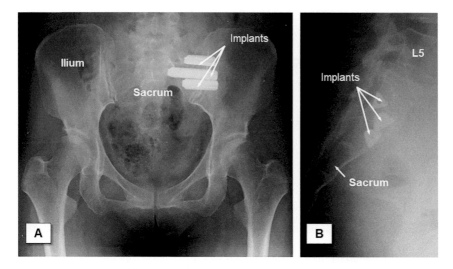

Figure 5.12 Lateral approach. Post-surgical images of the implants in the anterior (A) and mediolateral (B) views.

via the wires at the desired length. Finally, using the same technique, a third implant is inserted at a more caudal position in the joint so that the joint is fixed at three points.

5.4.3   Associated Risks

In both triangular titanium implant and screw placement, risks associated may include trauma to branches of the superior gluteal artery, hematoma, infections, screw dislocation, or loosening, especially in osteoporotic patients, damage to the L5 nerve root at the upper rim of the sacral ala, and perforation into a sacral neuroforamen.

5.5   Pitfalls of Sacroiliac Joint Arthrodesis in Patients with Sacral Dysmorphism

by Daisuke Kurosawa

Lumbosacral transient vertebrae can cause sacral dysmorphism combined with sacroiliac articular morphological changes. There are several technical pitfalls when performing sacroiliac joint arthrodesis in patients with sacral dysmorphism induced by lumbosacral transient vertebrae. A surgical plan should be made, including surgical approaches, while considering the type of sacral dysmorphism in each lumbosacral transient vertebrae type (Figure 5.13) (Kurosawa et al., 2020).

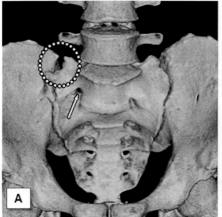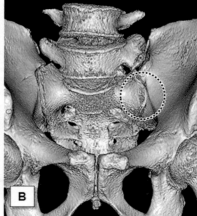

Figure 5.13 Sacral dysmorphism induced by lumbosacral transient vertebrae. (A) In Castellvi's Types II and IV, most cranial sacrum foramina are larger and irregularly round on the diarthrodial side (white arrow). The cranial sacral body (sacral alar) is thinner than usual when patients have any type of LSTV except for Type I (white dotted circle). (B) In Type I, the sacrum becomes small when the S1 vertebra appears like a lumbar vertebra (black dotted circle).

References

Ashman B, Norvell D, Hermsmeyer J (2010) Chronic sacroiliac joint pain: fusion versus denervation as treatment options. *Evidence-Based Spine-Care Journal*, **1**, 35–44.

Bai Z, Gao S, Liu J, Liang A, Yu W (2018) Anatomical evidence for the anterior plate fixation of sacroiliac joint. *Journal of Orthopaedic Science*, **23**, 132–136.

Booth J, Morris S (2019) The sacroiliac joint—victim or culprit. *Best Practice & Research in Clinical Rheumatology*, **33**, 88–101.

Dengler J, Kools D, Pflugmacher R, Gasbarrini A, Prestamburgo D, Gaetani P, Cher D, Van Eeckhoven E, Annertz M, Sturesson B (2019) Randomized trial of sacroiliac joint arthrodesis compared with conservative management for chronic low back pain attributed to the sacroiliac joint. *Journal of Bone and Joint Surgery*, **101**, 400–411.

Forst SL, Wheeler MT, Fortin JD, Vilensky JA (2006) The sacroiliac joint: anatomy, physiology and clinical significance. *Pain Physician*, **9**, 61–68.

Fuchs V, Ruhl B (2018) Distraction arthrodesis of the sacroiliac joint: 2-year results of a descriptive prospective multi-center cohort study in 171 patients. *European Spine Journal*, **27**, 194–204.

Galbusera F, Casaroli G, Chande R, et al. (2020) Biomechanics of sacropelvic fixation: a comprehensive finite element comparison of three techniques. *European Spine Journal*, **29**, 295–305.

Keating J, Dims V, Avillar M (1995) Sacroiliac joint fusion in a chronic low back pain population. In *The Integrated Function of the Lumbar Spine and Sacroiliac Joint, Part I*, pp. 361–365. Rotterdam: ECO.

Kurosawa D, Murakami E, Aizawa T, Watanabe T, Ozawa H (2020) Pitfalls during sacroiliac joint arthrodesis for patients with severe sacroiliac joint pain: report of three cases with sacral dysmorphism induced by lumbosacral transitional vertebrae. *Journal of Orthopaedic Case Reports*, **10**, 54–57.

Lindsey DP, Kiapour A, Yerby SA, Goel VK (2015) Sacroiliac joint fusion minimally affects adjacent lumbar segment motion: a finite element study. *International Journal of Spine Surgery*, **9**.

Martin CT, Haase L, Lender PA, Polly DW (2020) Minimally invasive sacroiliac joint fusion: the current evidence. *International Journal of Spine Surgery*, **14**, 20–29.

Murakami E, Kurosawa D, Aizawa T (2018) Sacroiliac joint arthrodesis for chronic sacroiliac joint pain: an anterior approach and clinical outcomes with a minimum 5-year follow-up. *Journal of Neurosurgery: Spine*, **29**, 279–285.

Polly DW, Cher DJ, Wine KD, et al. (2015) Randomized controlled trial of minimally invasive sacroiliac joint fusion using triangular titanium implants vs nonsurgical management for sacroiliac joint dysfunction: 12-month outcomes. *Neurosurgery*, **77**, 674–690.

Polly DW, Swofford J, Whang PG, et al. (2016) Two-year outcomes from a randomized controlled trial of minimally invasive sacroiliac joint fusion vs. nonsurgical management for sacroiliac joint dysfunction. *International Journal of Spine Surgery*, **10**, 28.

Schenker A, Schiltenwolf M, Schwarze M, Pepke W, Hemmer S, Akbar M (2019) [Pain generator sacroiliac joint: functional anatomy, symptoms and clinical significance]. *Der Orthopäde*, **49**, 1000–1005.

Schoell K, Buser Z, Jakoi A, et al. (2016) Postoperative complications in patients undergoing minimally invasive sacroiliac fusion. *The Spine Journal*, **16**, 1324–1332.

Schütz U, Grob D (2006) Poor outcome following bilateral sacroiliac joint fusion for degenerative sacroiliac joint syndrome. *Acta Orthopaedica Belgica*, **72**, 296–308.

Spain K, Holt T (2017) Surgical revision after sacroiliac joint fixation or fusion. *International Journal of Spine Surgery*, **11**, 5.

Vanaclocha V, Herrera JM, Saiz-Sapena N, Rivera-Paz M, Verdu-Lopez F (2018) Minimally invasive sacroiliac joint fusion, radiofrequency denervation, and conservative management for sacroiliac joint pain: 6-year comparative case series. *Neurosurgery*, **82**, 48–55.

Wise CL, Dall BE (2008) Minimally invasive sacroiliac arthrodesis: outcomes of a new technique. *Journal of Spinal Disorders and Techniques*, **21**, 579–584.

Yson SC, Sembrano JN, Polly DW (2019) Sacroiliac joint fusion: approaches and recent outcomes. *Physical Medicine and Rehabilitation*, **11**, S114–S117.

Index

Note: Numbers in *italics* indicate figures on the corresponding page.